Fitness for People with Disabilities

Fitness for People with Disabilities

Authors:
Matthew Witiw
Austin Mardon

Edited By
Riley Witiw
Catherine Mardon

Cover Design:
Josh Harnack

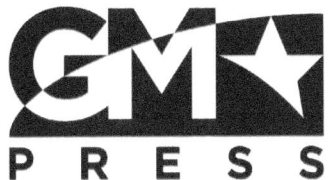

Copyright © 2022 by Austin Mardon

All rights reserved. This book or any portion thereof may not be reproduced or used in any manner whatsoever without the express written permission of the publisher except for the use of brief quotations in a book review or scholarly journal.

First Printing: 2022

Typeset and Cover Design by Josh Harnack

ISBN: 978-1-77369-781-9
E-Book ISBN: 978-1-77369-782-6

Golden Meteorite Press
103 11919 82 St NW
Edmonton, AB T5B 2W3
www.goldenmeteoritepress.com

Disclaimer

Although I have meticulously researched all the subjects I talk about and have personal experience in many of them, I am not a substitute for a healthcare professional. To be fair, that hasn't stopped Joe Rogan's 11 million listeners from taking what he says as law. Please question what I say and look into it yourself if you feel it necessary. Always consult a healthcare professional first when there is potential any activity I recommend may get you hurt.

Table of Contents

Introduction	9
Fitness with Disabilities	12
Mobility Issues	*12*
Cardiovascular Disease	*13*
Neurodegenerative Diseases	*13*
Final Word	*14*
Tips to Commit to Making a Change	15
General Principles of Diet	21
Dieting – Specific Circumstances	27
i- Dieting While Exercising	*27*
ii- Fad Diets	*32*
iii- Dieting with Cardiovascular Disease	*33*
iv- Dieting and Neurodegenerative Disease	*35*
v- Conclusion	*36*
General Principles of Exercise	37
i- Resistance Training as a form of Exercise	*40*
ii- Other Forms of Exercise	*50*
Exercising – Specific Circumstances	52
i- Exercise for People with Mobility Issues	*52*
ii- Exercise for People with Cardiovascular Disease (Interview with an Exercise Physiologist)	*55*
iii- Exercise for People with Neurodegenerative Diseases	*64*
Starting your Exercise Program	68
i- Resistance Training at the Gym	*68*
ii- Resistance Training from Home	*70*
iii- Other Forms of Exercise	*71*
Interview with a Success Story	76
i- Catherine Mardon	*76*
ii- Catherine on Exercise	*77*
iii- Catherine on Diet	*80*
iv- The Mind Games	*82*
v- Keep it Light-Hearted	*85*
Take that First Step, and the Next one…	87
Chapter by Chapter References	89

Introduction

Let's just face it, staying fit is hard. One week of exercise and healthy eating can quickly be derailed by grandma's famous cabbage rolls and butter encrusted pierogis. After eating a copious amount of this delicious food, the impending food coma might just make you sleep through the exercise time you had planned. Alright, I'll admit that was a pretty specific example. Still, the point is that everybody has their weaknesses that disrupt their fitness goals.

Unfortunately for some people, this fitness barrier seems, or is, more significant than for others. Many people have to deal with disabilities that may reduce the number of exercise programs that apply to them. Many fitness influencers stress how important and easy it is to be in shape, but their fitness routines are inaccessible for any beginner, let alone a beginner with a disability.

A quick introduction to myself: Hi, I'm Matthew, the awkward author who rants about pierogi and cabbage rolls. Why should you listen to anything a skinny 24-year old has to say about fitness, you ask? Well, that's a good question. My background is a bachelor's of science in pharmacology, so not precisely related to fitness. I played some high school basketball and football but certainly wasn't a sporting prodigy. I have no physical or mental disabilities that make fitness more challenging.

To those who still haven't thrown the book away, thanks! I will get to why you should definitely read this book, despite my background that may not feel directly relevant. I thought it necessary to specify that I've never come across many of the challenges people with disabilities face, and much of the research I have done was on my own time and not through a school program. As such, I haven't undertaken all of the fitness routines that I will write about in this book. However, the content I discuss in this book is well researched and includes interviews with people with unique and relevant perspectives. In addition, fitness is an integral part of my own life and something that I have a passion for. During my schooling, I learned how to accurately appraise research papers and sources of information to determine which information was well researched and which was not. I've combined my research skills, passion for fitness, and network of people with knowledgeable fitness perspectives to help people with disabilities on their own fitness journeys.

So what exactly have you got yourself into? What is this book about? What exactly is fitness?

Fitness is a term that can mean many different things to different people. People will have divergent views of who is physically fit and who isn't. Since it is a matter of perspective, you first have to define what it means to you. For me, fitness means having a healthy heart, going on long hikes with ease and being, as my brother calls it, skinny-jacked. To others, it may mean being as healthy as possible, walking for 15 minutes, or bench pressing 225 lbs. Take a second to define what it means to you right now.

While this definition has to primarily come from yourself, I have a few suggestions for defining fitness. First and foremost, fitness should be healthy. You should actively work on having a healthy heart. Cardiovascular diseases are very prevalent and dangerous. Not only will having a healthy heart make you live a longer life, but it will also improve your quality of life. However you define fitness, it will likely be a combination of diet and exercise that will get you there.

This book will begin by explaining general rules for dieting and exercise and how they pertain to people with disabilities. As many of you have probably already begun to suspect, there's no way I can cover every single disability that affects fitness in-depth in this book. First of all, I will note that I will predominately cover physical rather than mental disabilities. Even with this distinction, different physical disabilities affect people in totally different ways, so I've attempted to cover three prevalent categories: mobility issues, cardiovascular disease, and neurodegenerative diseases. I will also address what I think is the hardest part of fitness: committing to change. To paraphrase Newton's first law, a body at rest will remain at rest, and a body in motion will remain in motion. Sure, I'll admit, Isaac Newton meant this purely for physics, and he's probably rolling in his grave hearing it used like this. Still, I believe it rings true in many parts of life.

Great things begin with just a small step in the right direction. For example, starting to exercise. There's quite a lot to know before you start so you can do it safely and correctly. It can seem like a very daunting task. Another example was writing this book. Where do I start? How do I decide what to talk about? Once you start going, however, you realize it's much simpler than you had built it up to be. This principle also applies to people with disabilities. You just have to focus on what you can do rather than what you can't.

After taking that first step, the next section of this book will offer suggestions that make it easier to continue progressing and living your fit lifestyle. It's not an easy road ahead to be healthy and fit, especially if you have a disability, but it's entirely possible. In the final section, I'll drive this point home with an interview from a success story, Catherine Mardon, who suffered from being significantly overweight and having virtually no mobility.

By reading this book, you're already well on your way to taking

that first step. Let's get there together.

Fitness with Disabilities

I stated earlier that the three general categories of physical disabilities covered in this book are mobility issues, cardiovascular disease, and neurodegenerative diseases. What exactly does each of these categories mean? This chapter will answer that question and detail some of the unique problems these disabilities pose.

Mobility Issues

Mobility issues seem like a broad category, so what do I mean by this? The definition I'll be going by is straightforward: mobility issues are the impairment of one's ability to get around. The underlying cause of these issues is where it gets messy, though. These difficulties can be caused by many things, such as injuries, lack of fitness, ageing, neurodegenerative diseases and diabetes, among many others. Varying underlying causes mean that certain people will have lower mobility in the upper body in addition to the lower body.

Take, for example, ageing. As we get older, we have a more challenging time getting around and lose coordination and strength in our upper body. However, when I refer to mobility issues in this book, it means people who can't get around easily, while loss of upper body mobility is not implied. Still, people with upper-body mobility issues should find many of the general principles I discuss are relevant.

It may seem like the most prominent problem people with mobility issues face is how they ever do cardio. How can they do cardio if they can't do things like go on runs or walk on the treadmill? While they may look a little different, they absolutely can do cardio workouts. The general idea of cardio is getting your heart rate up through activity. While running and other activities where you're moving around are good cardiovascular workouts, they're not the only ones. There are plenty of ways to exercise and get your heart rate up without being on your feet.

Cardiovascular Disease

According to the World Health Organization (WHO), cardiovascular disease is the most common cause of death globally at a staggering 32% of all deaths. Cardiovascular diseases are a broad group of disorders that involve the heart or blood vessels. While cardiovascular diseases cause many deaths, most are not life-threatening with effective management. In fact, in most of my pharmacology classes, we didn't jump to hand out pills for cardiovascular disease. The first adjustment that should be made is in lifestyle. Eating healthy foods low in salt and engaging in regular activity are great ways to manage cardiovascular disease. That being said, there are varying types and severity of cardiovascular diseases, leaving much to be considered before diving headfirst into a very active lifestyle. For example, someone with a baseline high blood pressure must be careful not to raise their blood pressure too much, as it rises naturally while working out. This dichotomy will be further examined later in the book when I interview an exercise physiologist, Isaiah Stime. Despite these potential issues, there are ways to effectively exercise while mitigating these risks for people with cardiovascular disease.

Neurodegenerative Diseases

Neurodegenerative diseases involve the degeneration of the central and peripheral nervous systems. The most common are Parkinson's, Alzheimer's, and Huntington's disease. While there are often ways to slow the progression of these diseases or manage the symptoms, there is no known cure. This means that many of these diseases will result in progressive loss of muscle control and brain function. According to Nature, one of the world's leading research journals, one of the common pathologies of many neurodegenerative diseases is inflammation that ultimately results in adverse changes to the brain. Nature has published many recent papers that suggest that exercise reduces this inflammation in the brain and can reverse some of these effects. In addition, for diseases like Parkinson's with symptoms of tremors and rigidity, the Parkinson's Foundation suggests exercise as a way to combat these side effects. While exercise may be strenuous, especially as the disease progresses, maintaining an active training regime is more important than ever.

Final Word

Disabilities that may impede fitness come in all shapes and sizes, literally. The reality of writing this book is that I cannot address the specific issues with every type of physical disability. However, I will discuss the general principles of diet and exercise before addressing these particular ailments. Although this variety of disabilities may make it seem like most general fitness principles wouldn't apply, this isn't necessarily the case. The truth is that even though disabilities can limit some specific fitness routines, the general principles of dieting and exercising remain the same for everyone. That means that even if you have no disabilities or your disability is not in one of these three categories, this book will still have the knowledge to help you.

Tips to Commit to Making a Change

Whether you have a disability or not, you're going to need a spark to get you started on your fitness journey. You're also going to have to find ways to maintain and nourish that flame you began in the long term. This chapter will outline a simple three-step process to achieve these goals—a process that has been integral to my own fitness. The three-step process includes the first step, building a habit, and progression.

I can safely speak for most people when I say that we've all had those days when we think that we need to make a change and be more active. Unfortunately, a typical follow-up thought is, ehhh, I'll get started tomorrow. Then, we dive headfirst into another strangely binge-able Netflix series (seriously, are they developing some sort of evil algorithm to make these things impossible to stop watching?). The truth is, we often have seemingly lofty goals when it comes to our fitness—goals which are hard to motivate ourselves to achieve. For me, my initial plan was to build muscle from a skinny twig to being skinny-jacked. For somebody with obesity, it may be going from a place where they have nearly no mobility to running a marathon. When we think of the ultimate goals, they are often months or even years away. Hence, it is tough to commit to making that kind of change. Even if we undergo strenuous exercise and dieting for a few days or weeks to help achieve our goal quicker, our momentum can quickly be lost, leaving us right where we began. Here's the thing, sometimes a step in the right direction is even better than a leap.

Let's talk about that leap first. Something I've witnessed and struggled with myself in the past is what I'll call goal burnout. This happens when you have a lofty goal and go from doing nothing to achieve that goal to too much. In an ideal world, this would seem to make sense. The harder you work, and the more you do to reach a goal, the quicker you will achieve it, right? Well, yes, sort of. Everyone is different, and if you feel like you can do this, go for it and try it out! A word of warning, though, from what I've seen and done personally, most people burn hard and bright for a bit, maybe a month or so but then, they often burn out completely. I believe that this is because they go from something that takes no effort to maintain to something that takes lots of effort, and it's overwhelming. For some people, their goals will be less effort to them.

An example of this notion is people who love to train and exercise. Their genuine love for it helps them to maintain an active lifestyle. What about the people who want to be fit and don't necessarily enjoy doing it? Or the people who really enjoy food and it's a big part of their social life and interests? If that seems like you, there is no shame in it. I, for one, fit firmly into this category. Fitness still is very obtainable for people like us, but a leap into a super fit and healthy lifestyle is not the way to get there.

So what about that step? What if we take our ultimate goal and set up a series of sub-goals to reach it? What if instead of eating unhealthy every day of the week, we start by eating healthy just 1 day of the week? Sure, it will take longer to reach that ultimate goal of eating healthy and losing weight, but it is achievable, even for people who really like their pies. By setting up a series of smaller, more immediately achievable goals, we can find consistent feelings of accomplishment.

These first steps can be a wide variety of things: getting up and walking for ten minutes or doing stretches if you have mobility issues. If you are a person with a disability, it could even be getting health and fitness recommendations from your doctor. It could be doing ten minutes of research into a form of exercise or diet that may interest you. The important thing is that you're consistently setting a small amount of time aside to achieve this goal. It's the first part of my three "step" process (get it??).

The joke aside, the second and third parts of the three-step process should be done somewhat simultaneously. The second step is building a habit, and it's what makes leaping into fitness habits so tricky compared to taking small steps. Everyone has both good days and bad days when it comes to productivity. When people decide to make a leap, it is often on their good days when they feel productive. That's great, and maybe even a few more good days will roll by where they continue to rush towards their goal. However, there will be bad days that rear their ugly head—for leapers and steppers alike. Days when being productive seems like a monumental task. These days make it easy to fall off track and lose your momentum. When the bad days inevitably arrive, leapers will find it more challenging to overcome than steppers. In the early stages, motivating yourself is much easier if it's for a few small steps because your goal is more easily achievable. Also, you have much less momentum to lose in worst-case scenarios where you cannot motivate yourself. Hence, it is not as deflating to start again and easier to pick up where you left off. This means that you are more likely to continue over a long period with the three-step process. After a few months of consistently achieving your goals (though the exact length of time will vary amongst individuals), you begin to make a habit of it.

Awesome! So now you've formed your habit, that means it's easy to maintain and won't really take any effort, right? I hate to be the bearer of bad news, but I don't think easy will ever be the right word for living a healthy lifestyle. Having a habit is really great because it is more difficult to give up. For me, my habit of exercising means thinking of all the work I've put in how far I've come. The goals that I achieved have helped me live a more satisfying life, and I am unwilling to give that feeling of satisfaction up. When I am consistently not achieving my fitness goals, I feel unsatisfied. This quickly goes away when I start exercising again. Once you have a habit, when those blasted bad days come around and you can't muster up the motivation to achieve your goal, it will be much easier to start up again afterwards. Think of having a habit as having a constant baseline rate of momentum.

Finally, let's talk about the third step, progression, remembering that it should be done simultaneously with building a habit.

Progression is advancing towards a goal you have set. While forming a habit gives you the baseline momentum to keep working to achieve your goal, progression will make you see and feel the results. It does not necessarily have to be quick, but it must be consistent and lead towards your goals. There will be days when you will be physically unable to progress, and that is okay. Don't be frustrated—it's normal and happens to everyone. As long as you are actively attempting to progress and aren't just content with staying where you are, you will tend to move towards your goal.

One critical part of progression is tracking that progression. My goal to put on muscle was put on hold for years because I didn't track my progress. Instead of increasing the intensity of my workouts over the years, I found that I was simply content to do the same exercises and lift the same weights repeatedly. This may work okay for maintaining your current state, but you will not progress towards your ultimate goal. One day, after an intense workout with a friend, I lay gasping for air after our exercise routine. I looked up to see my friend looking nearly completely fresh—almost like he was ready for another exercise. How could he be that much more fit than I when we had been exercising for roughly the same timeframe? When I got up (with minor difficulty) and walked over, he was logging our workout in a small notebook. When I asked him about it, he explained that if you are serious about reaching a goal, tracking the progress is a near must. He simply progressed a little each exercise to get to where he was. When he forgot what he had done in previous exercises, he would merely look at what he had recorded in the notebook. It took him no more than a couple minutes to write it down. Depending on your goal, tracking progress can look very different, but I'd highly recommend that you write it down somewhere. It is too easy to forget exact details and misremember to keep track in your head, which can really impede you from accomplishing a long-term goal.

Taking the first step, building a habit, and progression. These are the parts of the three-step process, so what do they look like in action? Let me give an example. Let's say there is a particular red lightsaber-wielding person who recently underwent a tragedy.

They lost their legs and received severe burns due to having the low ground (I'm so sorry if you haven't watched Star Wars). They quickly received prosthetic legs, but losing their legs and other circumstances in their life were very hard on them mentally. Over the next few years, they put on a lot of weight and were rarely physically active. This went on until one day when they decided they needed to be more physically healthy to do their job well (intergalactic domination). Having read this book and knowing about the three-step process, they decided to take a step and make a change.

First, they contacted their doctor and told them about their plans to increase their fitness. The doctor suggested that they started by eating healthier and referred them to a physiotherapist to give them a proper exercise regime. This may seem like an easy thing to do, and that's just perfect. It was the first step in their fitness journey. Unfortunately, having recently spent all of his galactic credits on respiratory equipment, this individual wouldn't be able to afford a physiotherapist in the long term. To compromise, they decided that they would go once every couple of months to let a health expert check in on them. They told their physiotherapist about their issue and that they would only be back once every couple of months. The physiotherapist was understanding and showed them an exercise regime that they could do with their limited mobility. In addition, having read the next chapter of this book about diet, they decided to eat healthy three days a week and portion control the unhealthy foods they ate. They felt that this would be very achievable for them and a comfortable place to start dieting. Remember, everyone's starting point is different. A good starting point toes the line between pushing you and overwhelming you.

Now continuing with the story, it was time for steps two and three, building a habit and progression. For two weeks, they ate healthy three days of the week and portion controlled unhealthy foods every day. To track their results, they simply wrote on a calendar if they had eaten healthy that day or not. One day, they did not portion control their unhealthy food, and they also recorded this. They understood that everyone has slip-ups and simply recovered by continuing their usual routine afterwards.

They did this for two weeks and decided to begin with their first progression step, increasing the number of healthy days they ate to four. Over the next two weeks (weeks three and four), they found that they had lost weight. After the fourth week, the next step of progression was to start their exercise regime. They began by exercising for 30 minutes three days a week and recording the results. They continued to increase their daily exercise by five minutes every week until they reached one hour of activity in a single day. At this point, they were eating healthy four days per week, portion controlling the unhealthy food they ate, and exercising three days per week. This is where I'll end this example, but it could either continue going or not since fitness is subjective.

You may have noticed that choosing what to progress is subjective. Instead of increasing the amount of time worked out each session, you could also increase the number of days per week that you exercise. The critical thing is progressing by increasing the total amount of intensity you are putting in per week. I will dive into what intensity means in the chapter on general exercise. So what happens once you reach your initial ultimate goal? Hopefully, when you get to your initial ultimate goal, you will realize that you have made a complete lifestyle change. Maintaining your current fitness should be much easier, and you have the experience to set and work towards new goals.

Of course, everybody is different. The three-step method won't be the best way to get results for everyone. Some people are leapers and can quickly jump into significant lifestyle changes. Others may need to find different methods to commit to making a change. It is essential to be honest with yourself. Who would know best if a particular approach to commit and maintain a change in your life would work for you? You would. Try different things out, read about methods to motivate yourself. It is rarely easy to make this change, but anything is possible if you are genuinely willing to commit to making the change.

General Principles of Diet

Here it is again, another person telling you to eat healthily and making it sound easy as pie to have no pie. Let's be honest though, it's not. Eating foods can not only be enjoyable, but it can also be a large part of our social lives. Not only do many holidays often involve some sort of sinfully delicious feast, but even meeting up with friends for some food at a restaurant is a good way to stay in contact. This is all to say I understand that it is difficult and I think eating perfectly all the time has its drawbacks.

However, dieting properly can help you lose weight, and getting the nutrients you need makes you feel good and healthy. When people are struggling with weight or cardiovascular issues, jumping right into an exercise regime can be very difficult. A great first step is to begin dieting and losing weight, increasing the number of exercises these people can do. Further, when exercising, dieting properly can have a synergistic effect that helps you achieve your goals much quicker than you would otherwise.

So, in summary, I have reflected on the difficulty and potentially detrimental impacts of dieting. Conversely, I have also stated the importance of dieting in a healthy life. For those of you who read that and think to yourselves, it sounds doable, great! Some people can live very happily while adhering to diets nearly perfectly. Still, I believe that many people are unable to do this. If you cannot, that's alright—neither can I. The solution, as always, is a compromise. Understanding the principles of dieting and healthy eating lets you judge if you are swinging too far into unhealthy eating or eating healthy with absolutely no exceptions.

Let's start with some tips from the Canadian food guide on eating healthy in general. If you are interested in dieting, I would recommend checking out the Canadian food guide website yourself, as it offers some great diet tips and advice on how to eat healthily. They recommend ensuring that you have three meals a day while limiting snacks in between. This is important for a couple reasons. Firstly, it reduces the amount of binge eating you do. The longer you go without eating, the more hunger hormones you will produce. Consequently, you will likely end up eating the same amount even if you have two meals a day because you will be more hungry when you finally eat. Having three meals means that your hunger hormones will peak lower because there is less time between meals. The hunger hormones are obviously not very pleasant, and it is much more comfortable when they are stable. Having three meals a day will keep your hormone levels balanced and you happy. Limiting snacks is helpful because they are tricky to track, and you will likely underestimate how much you ate. Unfortunately, it is too easy to let snacking get out of hand, and when it does, it can derail what was otherwise a very healthy day of eating. If snacks are a must, try to ensure most of them are healthy, like vegetables or unflavoured yogurt with a bit of honey in it. Better yet, track your snacks so you know exactly what you have eaten. If you stick to these two rules, you will stabilize your hunger levels and eat a more consistent amount.

Now, for the compromise part of this rule. A life without the occasional unhealthy snacks sounds pretty tough, especially if you are just going cold turkey. It is entirely normal to have an off day, whether you planned it around a holiday or it was a spontaneous one that came out of nowhere. These days are sometimes necessary, and you shouldn't feel bad for having them! If you accept that you will have them, it is easier to plan around them to bounce back. My recommendation is to eat healthy five out of seven days of the week. This way, you are eating healthy most of the time, with a bit of flexibility. On your off days, ensure you are still utilizing portion control.

Portion control is my biggest recommendation to anyone who wants to lose weight, gain weight, or just eat generally healthy. Portion control is actively monitoring your food intake to know you are eating a proper amount of food. It applies to both healthy and unhealthy foods on your off days and ensures that you don't overeat or undereat. Depending on your current size and goal, portion control varies significantly between individuals. Consequently, giving a specific amount you should portion control for is difficult. An excellent way to measure the amount you are eating is through calories. Your age, sex, weight, and height will affect what is called your basal metabolic rate, the number of calories your body is burning each day for vital functions. In addition to this, your activity levels also affect the number of calories you should be ingesting. There are many calorie counters online, but I recommend asking your doctor or personal trainer what your caloric intake should be considering your goals. Once you find the number of calories you should be ingesting per day, divide that amount by three, and you will know exactly what you should be shooting for per meal. You will want to measure your food out the first few meals and make sure the calories line up. A helpful trick is to use the same size of plates and bowls so you begin to remember how much of your dishes should be covered up. As you get used to eating that amount, it will not be necessary to measure precisely, and you will begin to take much less time to prepare your meals. To reduce the time you take making meals initially, try meal prepping. Meal prepping is cooking a meal in bulk and storing it so you can quickly whip up a few portion-controlled meals throughout the coming days or weeks.

Now that you have a basic understanding of portion control, let's talk about what kind of food should be filling that plate. There are specific kinds of food to avoid for certain people, such as people with cardiovascular issues, which I will discuss later. I will start by just giving a general guide for everyone. Once again, I will quote what the Canadian food guide has to say.

Let's start with drinks. There are so many delicious drinks, but unfortunately, they are delicious for a reason. Drinks are often packed with so many sugars they will take up a disproportionate amount of your daily calorie count. The quality of the sugars is also suspect and usually bad for your health. One of the most consistent and vital recommendations is that water should be your drink of choice, basically all the time. Water fulfills the fundamental purpose of drinks, which is to quench your thirst without adding any additional calories to your diet. I know many people close to me who really don't enjoy having water and love other drinks, like iced tea, for example. So let's talk about that compromise once again. Be real with yourself—if you feel like sugary drinks are something you could easily cut out, then do it. But if they're not, consider drinking 350ml of whatever you want per day, and then switching back to water. This is likely limiting many calories, sodium, or sugars you were ingesting before while allowing yourself a solid taste of that drink you really enjoy.

Now, exactly how much water should you be drinking per day?

It's a surprisingly controversial question. I have met people who believe that there is a specific amount you should drink per day that is tons. In fact, I remember from when I was a kid that the Canadian food guide said eight cups per day. I'm going to be honest with you guys, though. This is an oversimplified answer. There are tons of variables that will affect the amount you should drink to stay hydrated. For most people though, the answer is actually quite simple. As my physiology professor quite eloquently put it: when you are thirsty, drink. Given that hydration is absolutely essential, our bodies are pretty good at telling us when we need water. Often, people are dehydrated because they are a little thirsty, but water is not readily available, meaning they would have to walk across the house to get it. My recommendation here would be to bring a water bottle with you wherever you go. This way, this won't be a cause for dehydration. There are also people whose bodies are not great at telling them when they are thirsty, which is a clinical condition. These people should obviously disregard this rule and drink a specific amount.

With drinks out of the way, let's talk about what should be on that plate. The Canadian food guide suggests that half of your plate be filled with vegetables. These will give you fibres, vitamins, and nutrients that you will simply not get in your diet without vegetables. Next, they suggest filling a quarter of your plate with protein of some sort, emphasizing having fish a couple times per week because it is vitamin and mineral-rich. Protein is a vital nutrient for your muscles and bones, but remember, it doesn't only come from meats. There are advantages and disadvantages of different forms of proteins, but the crucial part for most people is just having it in their diets. Beyond this, plant-based proteins can have more fibres and less saturated fats, which can be beneficial. If you have specific dietary needs, you should speak to a doctor or specialist about which forms of protein you should seek out or avoid. Finally, they recommend filling the last quarter of your plate with whole-grain foods such as whole grain rice, pasta, and quinoa. These foods contain carbohydrates for your energy and contain fibre and other healthy stuff that you won't get in the non-whole grain forms.

Straying from this very specific eating regime is okay too! Just be aware that you should do your best to include these food groups as often as possible to get a spread of the nutrients you will need. Now, you should be mindful that the foods you should avoid are just as important as those you should consume. Foods that contain lots of sugars, saturated fats, and sodium should be avoided—ingredients often contained in highly processed foods.

Let's talk about fats. There are several different types of fat that differ by molecular structure. While our bodies burn them all for fuel and various other uses, they have different effects on our bodies. According to Harvard University, the type of fat you should avoid the most is trans fats. Trans fats don't have the same benefits as other fats, but they certainly have a lot of harmful effects on your cholesterol levels and heart. In fact, there have been many efforts in Canada to limit the use of trans fats, and it is a lot less widely available than it has been in the past. Still, always look at your foods and make sure they have no trans fats. Since there are many alternative options, I would recommend that trans fats be an area where you try not to compromise and avoid them at all costs.

Saturated fats can be used for our bodies and are beneficial in moderation. Even then, according to Canada's government website, more than half of Canadians already have too many saturated fats in their diets. On the other hand, Harvard University refers to a meta-analysis (a collection of studies reviewed by experts in the field) that suggested saturated fats may actually not be as bad as previously thought. Still, there are benefits towards looking at the third, good kind of fat.

Unsaturated fats are what you should aim at getting in your diet. Ultimately, some fats are essential for your diet, but unsaturated fats are the best choice, given their benefits for cholesterol and reducing the risk of heart disease.

If you weaponize this information, your health will improve significantly. Remember that you will likely have days that you eat very unhealthy—again, that's okay. Always aim to eat healthy the majority of the time, but recognize you are a human with other aspirations and feelings other than your ultimate goal of fitness. These should be nourished while also generally moving towards your fitness goal.

Dieting – Specific Circumstances

Now that we've explored what a typical diet should look like, this chapter will address specific dietary recommendations. Some situations will call for an alteration in your diet or limiting particular substances. I will talk about dieting while exercising, fad diets, and dieting with cardiovascular or neurodegenerative diseases. If a certain section here doesn't interest you, just skip through it. I'll even give the different sections headlines for your skipping pleasure!

i- Dieting While Exercising

Dieting while exercising is essential for those who want to lose, gain, or maintain a specific weight. Often, people exercise because they want to lose weight or gain muscle mass. They misunderstand that a proper diet is imperative to fulfill those goals. Exercising and dieting have a synergistic effect on weight transformations. While dieting alone can help you lose weight, exercising will burn additional calories, making it much easier to lose weight. For muscle building, results hinge on a resistance training regime combined with the proper diet. Ultimately if you are putting in the hard work of exercising, dieting is still a must to achieve substantial results.

When exercising, you should adhere to the general principles for eating healthy and portion sizes for food groups. However, there are additional nutrient and calorie requirements to consider depending on your goals. I will discuss a few general situations and what nutrients you should uptake to make those goals a reality.

First of all, if your goal is to lose weight, there are a few things to consider. In general, you should always maintain a slight caloric deficit. If you recall from earlier, I discussed how you have a basal metabolic rate, meaning your body burns a certain amount of calories a day as a baseline. When you are active, you burn additional calories on top of your basal metabolic rate. Use one of the methods discussed earlier to calculate your basal metabolic rate. You'll also want to have a way to track the approximate amount of calories that you are burning during activity. Some devices like the Apple watch calculate a rough estimate of this for you. In addition, an online search like "how many calories does a 20-minute run burn?" is also a way to figure out an approximation. It is okay that these are not precise measurements, as the rough estimate should give you a general idea.

A caloric deficit means taking in fewer calories than you have burnt in a day. You can determine the amount of calories you have burnt in a day by adding your basal metabolic rate to the calories burnt from your activities. To have a caloric deficit, the number of calories you consume should be less than your total calories burnt in a day. So if you want to lose a lot of weight, you should have a large caloric deficit, right? Wrong. It is crucial to ensure that your caloric deficit is not too much because calories are needed for survival. They provide the body with the necessary energy to properly function. A good calorie deficit for losing weight is between 500 to 1000 calories per day. Personally, I would suggest a 500 calorie deficit because, over time, this amount will still effectively help to reduce weight and is more manageable long-term. While different food groups like vegetables and grains should still take up the same proportion of your plate, you need to ensure you get your protein and carbohydrates. This focus on protein and carbohydrates when you are frequently exercising gives you energy and helps you repair and build muscle damaged during exercise.

Now let's talk about if your goal is losing weight while putting on muscle. First and foremost, this is a very challenging goal to obtain. People who are just beginning to diet and exercise will find it much more achievable than people with high muscle, low fat physiques. You will need to remain patient and remember that this is a lifestyle change and won't happen overnight. The principles I talk about here are the same as they are for "cutting," which means keeping muscle mass while losing fat. For most people, a resistance training routine will be much more successful than general exercise to gain significant amounts of muscle mass. Like the general principle of losing weight, you will want to have a slight caloric deficit of 500 calories per day. I would not suggest a 1000 calorie per day deficit because there will be additional nutrients you will need to consume because you are trying to build muscle. Whenever your goal is to increase muscle mass, you will need to take up extra protein in your diet. The American College of Sports Medicine recommends those in resistance weight training programs take up 1.2 to 1.7g of protein per kg of bodyweight. In other words, you should take 0.5 to 0.8g of protein per pound of body weight per day. For example, a 200 lb individual should be taking up about 100-160 g of protein per day if they wish to gain muscle mass.

The American College of Sports Medicine also states that you should be able to uptake this amount of protein in a regular diet without protein supplements. While this assertion is true in theory, it's hard to take up that much protein! I often spend a long time surveying the protein content of different foods in the grocery store, wondering why the human body finds the need to make everything so darn difficult. Trying to get all that protein while on a caloric deficit, you will need to find high protein foods that are also low on calories. There is lots of protein to be found, though, and after a couple times in the grocery store, you find foods that are high protein that you enjoy and can continue to eat for a long time. What comes to my mind is the old chicken breast and rice diet. While I can't say I'd appreciate that, some people really do! If that doesn't float your boat, since protein is easy to find in many foods, even people who crave variety in their meals should be able to have it.

Another mentionable thing about protein is that the timing matters. The American College of Sports Medicine relates that taking up protein before or up to an hour after a workout may have additional muscle building and recovery benefits. However, you should be careful in overeating before a workout, so you don't cramp up. I would suggest having one of your meals soon after your workout. It can really make everything worthwhile once you start seeing those hard-earned results. This notion especially applies when trying to lose weight while gaining muscle. Progress may be slow, but the long-term results are highly satisfying.

Another nutrient that is important if you exercise and want to gain muscle is carbohydrates. Carbohydrates are essential because your body will use them for energy instead of protein. You need that protein in your body to build muscle. It will also give you the energy to improve your performance while working out, increasing your muscle gain. The American College of Sports Medicine cites this energy requirement at an additional 60 to 90g of carbs per hour of intense exercise. While there are many different forms of carbohydrates, be careful because they can push that calorie count up quick! Rice is a good option for carbs because it is relatively lower in calories than other options. Brown rice, in particular, is a great choice. Not only is it low in calories, but it also contains other vital nutrients like fibre. Beyond diet and resistance training, the most challenging thing about gaining muscle while losing weight is the time it takes. It really is a marathon, not a sprint. That being said, it is entirely possible as long as you really put the effort in.

The third goal I wanted to discuss is solely focusing on building muscle. This is what is often referred to as a "bulk." This method will be the most effective in gaining muscle mass, but you will likely put on other weight as well. Of course, the more healthy you eat during your bulk, the less fat you will put on, making it essential to know your goals going into this method. If you are light and want to or need to put on weight, bulking is a great way to do so, but keep in mind that it's not a license to disregard your health.

You should typically have a slight calorie surplus of about 500 calories per day during a bulk. A calorie surplus means taking up more calories than your basal metabolic rate and calories burnt during activities combined. You may be tempted to eat unhealthy to consume all of these calories, but I would strongly suggest a healthy, balanced diet. Most people want to work out to stay fit, and if you are eating unhealthy just to gain muscle, you are actively doing the opposite. Eating unhealthy can cause latent cardiovascular issues and put on fat that will be difficult to lose later in life. There is also your body's basic anatomy to consider. I know people who used to be extremely muscular but developed knee and back problems later in life from the heavy lifting and carrying so much weight around every day. Be sure of your end goal. I believe there is a good balance here where you can put on muscle while also enduring a healthy lifestyle that will make you feel better now and in the future.

In addition to this calorie surplus, you should also have a protein uptake of 1.2 to 1.7 g per kg of body weight, or 0.5 to 0.8 g per lb. This intake should be done while maintaining your healthy eating proportions. Make sure you're still getting your vegetables and other nutrition while focusing on this goal. Again, there may be additional benefits to consuming this protein before or just after a workout and eating 60 to 90g of carbs per hour of intense exercise. This additional carbohydrate requirement can easily be met within your calorie surplus. Many options, such as multi-grain rice and potatoes, are healthy for you while fulfilling these requirements.

The last thing to mention in this section is dieting to maintain muscle. This process is best for people exercising for cardiovascular and mental health reasons with no weight goals. Take up about 0.8 g per kg of body weight, or about .36 g per lb, to maintain muscle. If you are 50 or above, this requirement is a bit higher, and you should take up about 1g per kg of body weight, or 0.45 g per lb. With this protein requirement in mind, you should still be free to focus on eating healthy, as discussed in the general diet section. The calories you consume should be near the number of calories you burn each day and still take up about 60 to 90g of additional carbs for each hour of intense exercise.

ii- Fad Diets

Fad diets are something that I learned a lot about in my pharmacology program. They are widespread, and some new diet is always emerging, with people claiming that it works great for them. They are so numerous that it makes it challenging to address them specifically, so I'll refer to all fad diets as a group here. However, that may not be entirely fair. A fad diet is any diet that becomes very popular for a short period. The inherent problem with fad diets is they are subject to varying amounts of research. I'll be referring to what is generally true for most of these diets.

Firstly, I strongly suggest portion control and proper nutrition for weight loss. In most cases, this method will work very effectively. As discussed in the previous chapter, the balanced nutrition you receive in a complete diet has been well researched to be very healthy for you in the long term. Fad diets such as keto, raw food, paleo, and the like may be okay if done correctly—emphasizing the may. I say this because I have not done very much personal research on these specific diets and don't know the extent of research. Some fad diets end up being wholly reasonable and healthy.

The main issue with fad diets is often a lack of research—specifically long-term studies. As a result of these diets popping up and promising quick results, they often blow up really quick. They have many people following them instantly, achieving the results they want. Unfortunately, significant research usually lags behind when these diets are already popular. Consequently, these diets could lack specific forms of nutrition or have harmful substances, or alternatively, nutrients that you are getting too much of. Essentially, the problem is that they are unknown.

If there were no other forms of weight loss, I think you could argue that it would be worth the risk, but this is why I strongly recommend portion control as a first step. At least see if it can work for you. If this methodology fails and you are interested in a fad diet, I would talk to a doctor or nutritionist about the diet that you are interested in. They will likely have heard of these popular diets or know people knowledgeable on the subject. Generally, asking a doctor is preferable because they are given the tools to understand research papers on the subject. I'm not saying that you cannot understand these papers yourself—just that doctors undergo years of rigorous schooling to accurately interpret findings. The bottom line is that you should really hear their perspective. Once you have gained your doctor's or nutritionist's perspective, choose whether the diet is right for you.

iii- Dieting with Cardiovascular Disease

One of the leading behavioural factors that cause cardiovascular disease is diet. That means that although it is difficult, it is imperative to improve your diet when dealing with cardiovascular disease or issues. Adhering to the general principles of diet will benefit most people with cardiovascular disease, but a highly researched diet exists specifically for cardiovascular disease.

The Dietary Approaches to Stop Hypertension, or DASH diet, was developed by the National Institute of Health. Hypertension is another word for high blood pressure—one of the most common risk factors for many different forms of cardiovascular disease. What differentiates this diet from fad diets is the amount of research done before it was available to the public. This information is all readily available online. You can read the separate studies, but experts have a very heavy consensus that this diet works. The diet helped to improve blood pressure and cholesterol in clinical trials. This may all sound very sciency and fancy, but one of the goals when designing this diet was to make it readily available to everyone. All of the needed ingredients can be obtained from your local grocery store. The general plan of this diet is to offer daily and weekly nutritional goals low in saturated fat, cholesterol, trans fat, and sugar-sweetened food. They accomplish this all while also having a balanced diet.

One problem with it being sciency is that it will take a bit of research and effort to maintain the DASH diet. Again, why does the human body need to make everything so complicated? It's ridiculous. Fortunately enough, we've already talked about some of the factors you need to consider when going on the DASH diet. Let's talk about the amount of food you would be eating. To assess the number of calories you need, you must consider your age, sex, and activity level.

A quick aside about sex here, typically XY chromosomes make the male primary and secondary sex characteristics (like male reproductive organs) beginning at birth. In contrast, XX chromosomes in your genetic code make female primary and secondary sex characteristics. They must test both in science because specific diets and other things will react differently between the sexes. There are, of course, exceptions (androgen insensitivity amongst others), so these are just general guidelines, don't feel like they must absolutely apply to you.

Typically, your body will burn fewer calories as you age, so you need to take up less. High activity levels will increase the number of calories you need in your diet. Biological males will also typically burn more calories than biological females. With these 3 factors taken into account, the DASH diet will assign a typical calorie marker you should be hitting each day. The DASH diet then takes this calorie level and assigns you a number of specific food servings relative to your calorie level.

The DASH diet emphasizes grains, vegetables, fruits, fat-free/low dairy products, lean meats, poultry, fish, nuts, seeds and legumes, and fats and oils. It will give you a number of servings for each of these food groups each day. For flexibility, the diet includes a sweets and sugars section, so you treat yourself within moderation. Another essential section of this diet is the maximum daily sodium limit it assigns you. Your sodium limit will change depending on the number of calories you should consume each day. This section is critical because excessive sodium is significantly detrimental to cardiovascular health.

The best part about the DASH diet is all the readily available information you can read about it. All the data is on the National Institute of Health web page about how they found out that it works, why it's effective, how to do it, and even tips to get started. If you are interested, search "DASH diet NIH" online. The diet is flexible by design, so although it takes some initial research, they have deeply considered what would make it a sustainable way of life. Ultimately, the DASH diet is an excellent option for individuals with cardiovascular issues.

iv- Dieting and Neurodegenerative Disease

Honestly, this section is not one I anticipated to include in this book. I didn't really believe that diet would benefit individuals with neurodegenerative diseases, such as Parkinson's and Alzheimer's. I was wrong. In my first few seconds of research, I discovered that specific diets may be able to reduce your chances of developing certain neurodegenerative diseases! This knowledge is particularly useful for people with risk factors associated with a neurodegenerative disease. An example of this is people with parents or grandparents who have heritable diseases. It's an exciting time, as research is rapidly developing in this area.

One study published in the American Journal of clinical nutrition by Gao et al. in 2007 found that a Mediterranean diet reduced the risk of developing Parkinson's later in life. I won't go too deep into the specifics about the Mediterranean diet here, but it has many fruits, vegetables, nuts, seeds, olive oil, and other whole grains. Are you noticing how many foods seem to repeat themselves in these highly researched diets?

Overall, the evidence does not definitively suggest that the Mediterranean or other diets will reduce the risk of Parkinson's or other neurodegenerative diseases. However, it will continue to be researched. You should pay attention to this research, especially if you know you have risk factors for any of these neurodegenerative diseases.

v- Conclusion

So I've now babbled on about general dieting principles, dieting while working out, fad diets, and dieting for cardiovascular and neurodegenerative diseases. Whether you have actually stuck with me through all of that or just skipped right through, I just wanted to leave you with one final take-home message. If you go all-in on a diet and burn yourself out, you will often get derailed and end up right back where you started. Improvement is absolutely key. As long as you consistently eat better until you reach your goal, you're doing great! Even if you're not seeing the immediate physical results you want, you are progressing by eating healthier, and the results will come. Just don't wait forever to take that first step. That damn body has a way of getting back at you for that.

General Principles of Exercise

We've now discussed committing to fitness and dieting—both integral parts of fitness—but maybe not what jumps to mind for most people when they think about fitness. Now let's talk about the big one: Exercise. How YOU can get SHREDDED in JUST 90 DAYS! Sounds too good to be true? Well, it is. The lifestyle adjustment alone from being unfit to extremely fit in 90 days alone would be too much to maintain. Fitness will be a long-term journey, but there are many routes you can take, and you might just find yourself a hobby you enjoy along the way. There are plenty of different forms of exercise, and it is really beneficial to find one that suits you well. This chapter will talk about various exercise forms and how to find the best one for you.

What exactly is exercise? According to the National Institute of Health, exercise is planned and structured physical activity. In contrast, physical activity is movement that is good for your physical health. Exercise mainly benefits from planning because you consistently do it, usually with a fitness-related goal in mind. Other forms of physical activity (going on walks etc.) can be inconsistent, and you can have bouts of not doing any activity at all. As we have discussed, this consistency helps you turn physical activity into a habit, which allows you to have a nice, healthy lifestyle.

Exercise benefits your heart in a multitude of ways. For example, it reduces your stress hormones while increasing mood-elevating hormones. Now, this concept may be a little misleading. At first, exercising can be really intimidating and challenging. Who goes into tough situations and thinks to themselves, "ah yes, so relaxing"? Nobody, that's who. Well, maybe that's an overgeneralization, so I'll just say most people wouldn't think that. Exercising is arduous and may not be relaxing for the first bit as you learn. Suppose you find a form of exercise you enjoy and make a habit of doing it. In that case, I promise that stress will fade and that beneficial body chemistry will start kicking in for you.

Another benefit of exercise is that it physically strengthens your heart if intense enough, making it work more efficiently. An efficient heart is less stressed and will operate for you better in the long term. An excellent way to measure the intensity of your exercise is to monitor your heart rate. The more intense the workout, the higher your heart rate will be. While exercising, you should aim to build up and maintain an elevated heart rate. If your exercise is not challenging enough for you, you will see this reflected in your heart rate, as it will not go as high. Conversely, some people, like those with cardiovascular issues, should be concerned with raising their heart rate too high. As a result, if you have any pre-existing cardiovascular problems, it is crucial to discuss heart rate goals with a medical professional. In the next chapter, exercise — specific circumstances, I interview an exercise physiologist, discussing heart rate goals in more depth. Exercising also lowers your risk of heart disease by reducing blood pressure in the long term and improving cholesterol, which lowers the resistance against your heart. Consequently, your heart's job gets a lot easier.

Beyond the beneficial effects of exercise on your heart, it also strengthens your muscles. This factor can help you choose which type of exercise you wish to pursue. Different activities will work your muscles to various degrees. Running primarily strengthens your legs, while proper resistance training builds your whole body. The activities you enjoy will also significantly affect the type of exercise you pursue. You might think it doesn't make much of a difference, but I believe it is absolutely the most critical factor in maintaining a fitness regime.

Imagine a person decides to do resistance training because they want to strengthen their whole body and look great. They work out four days a week for half a month, but really, they don't enjoy resistance training so much. Despite this disinterest, they are adamant that they want to look all muscly and nice, so they continue to work out. They already work a full-time job, and resistance training feels like an extra job, resulting in a strain on their mental health. Eventually, this strain causes them to fall off and stop working out altogether. Their lack of enjoyment makes it really hard to develop a habit, not to mention that having a routine you dread doing would be bad for your mental health.

But maybe not all is lost. Say this person really likes basketball. They join a men's league team that practices once per week and play a game every Saturday. This team provides an excellent baseline of two days a week of exercise that they actually enjoy. As a result of having fun, they can make playing basketball a habit and continue over the years—a habit that will bring them joy and improve their life. Still, while basketball is terrific for cardiovascular health, it does not help them meet their goal of putting on significant muscle mass. Once again, compromise can come to the rescue. Suppose they work out three days per week on top of playing basketball two days a week. In that case, they will be more likely to maintain this lifestyle while also reaching an important goal. Adding something you genuinely enjoy to your exercise regime is vital for long-term adherence to fitness and helps with mental health.

That's all fine and dandy if you enjoy a form of exercise, but what if you can't find an activity you like? Well, let's brainstorm here and try to come up with a compromise. I took a single first-year psychology course in school, so I'm pretty much an expert on motivation (right?). One idea is to hold off on a sedimentary activity you enjoy until you get your exercise in. Say you decide that you must exercise before doing your nightly Netflix binge. This may give you the drive to exercise consistently. If you think that abstaining from that Netflix binge will take too much willpower, ask somebody close to you to hold you accountable. Another idea would be to positively reinforce your exercise. Buy a chocolate bar and after each workout, have a piece of it. Just don't eat the whole thing—it could get out of hand pretty quick!

Another thing to make sure you're doing while exercising is hydrating. Hydration is critical, so always have a water bottle with you when you exercise. A tip I learned while playing sports is not to drink huge amounts of water all at once. This overindulgence can leave you feeling bloated and even increase your chances of puking. Gross!

Those were principles for exercises in general, but there are plenty of different forms of activities you can do to get in your exercise. All of these activities will have their own tips and tricks. The following sections will focus on different forms of exercise, with an extra emphasis on resistance training—something I have a fair amount of experience in.

i- Resistance Training as a form of Exercise

Resistance training is a superb form of exercise and likely has the most potential for extensive body transformations. Resistance training means using your muscles to work against a force. If one of your goals is increasing muscle mass, resistance training is your best bet to get those results.

Resistance training can look tremendously different based on your goals. Typically there are three types of intents: strength, muscle building (hypertrophy), and endurance training. If you want to work out for general fitness, I suggest endurance training because you will not be lifting as much weight. Therefore, there is less risk of injury. That being said, I personally resistance train for muscle building. As long as you are careful, any form of resistance training is a great exercise.

Strength training will be a good fit for you if you desire to get significantly stronger. That is not to say that muscle building and endurance training will not increase your strength. In fact, they certainly will. However, while the other forms of training will also increase your strength, it would not be to the same extent. An example of a goal you would set for strength training is, "I want to be able to squat x amount of weight."

Muscle building is excellent for people who want to increase their weight, decrease their fat while increasing muscle, or just look more muscular. Strength and endurance training will also help to build muscle, but muscle-building training is the most efficient in doing so. Of course, it should be noted that for these goals to be successfully completed, they will have to consider their diet, as stated earlier.

Muscular endurance may be the least enticing option, but it is probably the most practical for day-to-day life. It increases your muscles' ability to withstand force over a long period. Endurance training is excellent for sports performance, helps everyday posture, and offers a safer way to train where you are less likely to hurt yourself.

It should be noted that, although I will give general guidelines for these three resistance training goals, everyone is unique. What works for one person may not necessarily work for another because there are many variables such as age, sex, and your specific body. Beyond being patient and waiting for the results you want, if you feel like your training program is not working out as you want, try changing it up!

Remember earlier when I discussed planning and progression? Well, it is an absolute necessity when it comes to resistance training. If you go in without a plan, not only will you not get as high-quality of workouts, you are also likely to fall off and stop working out altogether. Before starting your resistance training, you're going to have to consider a few different factors that will affect your plan. The first one is frequency, or how often you're going to work out. Next, you must select the activities you will engage in during your workouts and how you will do them. Your end goals can help you decide on these two factors.

So let's talk about the first factor, frequency. How often should you work out? This number can vary between individuals, so don't feel like there is just one correct answer. Many sources I've read suggest three to six days per week of resistance training. What it's really going to depend on is your goals, though. Say you are doing resistance training to increase your fitness, with no muscle-building plans. In this case, you can factor in other activities like playing sports, going on walks, etc. and count them as workouts. An example of this is doing a full-body resistance training workout two times a week and running three times a week. However, there is strong evidence to suggest you should exercise each major body group two times per week to build strength and muscle. Consequently, if your goal is to build strength or muscle, you should be resistance training three to six times a week. Again, I'll say it for the 1000th time, nobody knows your situation better than yourself. If you are coming from a completely sedentary lifestyle, just getting out and training once or twice a week is an improvement, even if your end goal is muscle building. This regime is just your starting point. As long as you push yourself and progress to the point where you're working out three to six times a week, you'll eventually put on significant muscle. Keep pushing yourself!

So now that you know how frequently to work out when resistance training, the other factor is what you're going to do each day when you exercise. How are you going to split up your workouts? To decide this, you're going to need to know a bit of the underlying theory. Firstly, the body is usually divided into six or seven distinct muscle groups for planning resistance training workouts. These muscle groups are chest, biceps, triceps, back, shoulders, legs, and the seventh (sometimes not included) group: core. The core is not always considered, but that doesn't mean it's unimportant. The reason for the core's exclusion is because it's activated and strengthened while training many of the other muscle groups.

It's key to strengthen all seven of these muscle groups, or else you will end up with muscle imbalances. Countless memes have been created of the gym bro who skips leg day, but outside of people's relentless need to shame others, why is a muscle imbalance not good? Muscle imbalances can result in certain muscles overcompensating for the less developed muscles, increasing their risk of injury. That being said, it is acceptable to focus on specific muscle groups that you want to improve significantly. Just don't forget about the rest of your body as well.

When preparing your resistance training routine, I suggest planning the muscle groups you exercise based on the number of days you work out per week. Every week, you should plan on hitting each one of those body groups one to two days. Again, one day should be satisfactory for general fitness, but two days or more is necessary for muscle building. That means if you are resistance training two to three times per week, these workouts should likely be full-body workouts. If you plan on a more vigorous routine of five to six days per week, you can divide it differently. Picking two body groups from chest, biceps, triceps, back, shoulders and legs, with a small core component every day, is a great way to split it up. Another option is a four-day split where you exercise three body groups with a small core component each day.

You have flexibility when deciding which body groups to pair together. Often times chest is paired with triceps and shoulders since these muscles are often all utilized in the same resistance exercises. You will often hear these workouts called "push" days since many of the exercises that work these muscle groups involve pushing motions. Legs are often put on their own day because there are several muscles in the legs to be considered, such as quads, hamstrings, calves, and glutes. Biceps and back are then usually paired together. These are often called "pull" days since many workouts involve pulling motions. Obviously, there is a lot of variance in planning a resistance training regime. Depending on the number of days you work out, you could be pairing muscle groups together that I didn't suggest, and that's okay. This is just a general guideline that you should consider. Find a routine that works best for you and stick to it.

While these workout pairings focus on other body parts, you should never forget about your core or cardiovascular health when planning a resistance routine. You can pair core and cardiovascular health with other muscle groups—for example, having a core, back, and biceps day. Personally, I have found the most success doing a few core exercises each day. The same goes for your cardiovascular health. An indication of a good cardiovascular workout is a high heart rate, which means there are many ways to get to that endpoint. You can have a cardiovascular focus by running or simply having fast-paced workouts. Adults should aim to have a consistently high heart rate for about 150 minutes per week, while children and youth need about 60 minutes per day. Again, this goal is an endpoint. If you can't reach this optimal amount of minutes per week right off that bat, that's alright. In fact, immediately pushing yourself to this level right off the beginning is potentially dangerous. The overall idea is to work cardio and core into your resistance training routine.

So now I've gone over frequency and how you could split up workouts to strengthen your muscle groups evenly and effectively. Next, I'll discuss what to do each day you work out and suggest what your resistance routine could look like depending on your goals.

I find people forget that resistance training is ultimately about your physical health. Sure it's great to be strong and muscular, but what if you injure yourself badly? Depending on injuries severity, you could have to deal with it for the rest of your life. To me, it seems pretty counterproductive that you were doing all this work to improve your body just to end up harming it. That means that injury prevention should be a top priority. I'll talk about injury prevention throughout this section, starting with warming up before your workouts and cooling down after.

According to Harvard's medical school, you should aim to warm up for five to ten minutes before starting each workout. You may have heard that static (low movement) stretching is not great for a warmup. Well, the goal of the warmup should be getting your heart rate up to start circulating blood to all your major muscle groups. A static warmup will not get your heart rate up to where you want it to be. Cardio activities involve a full range of motion. Exercises like jumping jacks or even dancing are great for active warmups. Ensure that you are getting blood flow to all muscle groups in your warmup—even if you don't intend on exercising those specific muscles.

Cooling down after your exercise is also essential. It will also assist in injury prevention and will help gradually reduce your blood pressure, helping blood regulation and reducing stress on your heart. A successful cooldown consists of slow movements and static stretching. Cooldowns and warmups are critical for all forms of exercise, not just resistance training. As long as they are effective, you can use the same warmup and cooldown for resistance training as playing a basketball game.

Now finally, after a mere few paragraphs of ranting, I can get into the specifics of resistance training. Let's start out with the basics. When I say basics, I mean reaaalllly basic, then we can work up from there! First of all, let's talk about repetitions (reps), sets, and rest. They'll be important! Reps are the number of times you complete a particular exercise's full range of motion. For example, during a squat, getting down low and then going back up to your original standing position is a single rep of the exercise. A set is completing a certain amount of repetitions in a row without a break. The number of reps in a set will vary based on your goals, which I will discuss later in this section. In the context of resistance training, rest means taking a planned amount of time between each set of an exercise. It is essential to take rest time, but the exact amount of time again varies based on your goals.

Now that we've talked about the super basic stuff, let's get a little fancy. Let's talk about four different variations of sets: compound sets, supersets, circuits, and drop sets. All four of these set forms will have an additional cardio component and save you time during your workout if done with enough intensity. Compound sets are when you add two exercises of the same body group or non-opposing body groups back-to-back without a rest in between. You still take rest time, but only once both exercises are completed. This method will also fatigue your muscle quicker, which is ideal for muscle building and endurance training.

Next are supersets, often thought to be the same as compound sets. However, these two types of sets actually differ from each other! Like compound sets, you complete two exercises together in supersets. The important distinction is that the exercises work opposing muscle groups instead of the same muscle groups. An example would be a chest exercise combined with a back exercise or a bicep exercise with a triceps exercise. Supersets fatigue your muscle less than compound sets since your opposing muscle is resting while you do the other exercise and are generally better for strength training.

A circuit has a pretty straightforward definition—two or more of any exercise put together. Typically, you might lump three or four exercises together with a single rest period after completing them all. You can also mix and match whichever muscle groups in circuits. The main advantage of circuits is adding an additional cardio component to your set and decreasing your workout time. Your heart rate will remain high for an extended period, which is ideal.

Finally, there are also drop sets, which involve only one exercise. Essentially, you will start heavy and do as many repetitions as possible until failure. Aim for six to eight reps! Then, with no rest, you do a lighter weight for more reps and repeat this as many times as you want. This general format works if you have many different weights available to you, such as you would at a gym. That said, drop sets can still be helpful even if only a few weights are available. I use this type of set when I find one set of weights is too much for me, but the next weight below is too easy. For example, imagine you have two sets of dumbbells at 35 lb and 20 lb. The difference between the weights may be a significant drop-off in difficulty for many exercises. In this scenario, you should set a goal for how many reps you will do in your set. For example, aim to do 12 bicep curls. Then, do as many repetitions as you can at the high weight—hypothetically, let's say four reps at 35 lb. After, switch down to the weight below and finish the set. So, in this case, you would finish with eight reps of 20 lb, or until failure. Make sure that you minimize the amount of rest in between switching weight. Drop sets are not only helpful when fewer weights are available to you but are also great at fatiguing your muscles.

While these four sets are pretty similar, many workouts shake up the traditional format of doing a certain number of reps each set and resting before the next one. Examples include high-intensity interval training (HIIT) or as many reps as possible (AMRAP). My intentions for this chapter are to keep things pretty simple, so I won't go into depth on either. If you are interested in more advanced workouts like these methods, my advice would be to discuss them with a personal trainer or physiotherapist. They will have in-depth knowledge and guide you through these more complicated workouts.

Earlier in this chapter, I discussed resistance training goals like strength, hypertrophy, and endurance. The difference between these options is primarily the number of reps and sets you do. Strength training will have the lowest number of repetitions but the highest resistance. At the right weight, you should only be able to lift three to six reps for about two to five sets. You should also take larger rest times between sets of about two to five minutes. Giving your muscle time to recover reduces your muscles fatigue and allows you to lift as much weight as possible, which is key for strength training. Next is building muscle, where your goal is to fatigue the muscle rather than lift as much as possible. Fatiguing your muscle requires a combination of moderate resistance, as well as many repetitions to get your body's anaerobic energy system going. You should aim for eight to 12 repetitions and three to five sets for this goal. Your rest time should be less than strength-building—about 30 seconds to two minutes. For muscle endurance training, you should aim to do more than 12 repetitions for two to three sets. Rest time should be shortest here of about 20 to 30 seconds. Whenever you're lifting more weight, there's more of a risk of getting a severe injury. That's why if you're doing resistance training for general fitness reasons, I'd suggest starting with muscle endurance training.

While I may have made it sound like these rep and set ranges will definitely result in the desired goal, the exact numbers are often hotly debated. This discrepancy is because, in actuality, these ranges are flexible and fluid. If you go one repetition above or below, ultimately, it will not change your results much. My word is definitely not law, but the ranges I have given are a solid general guideline.

As far as specific exercises go, there are plenty for each muscle group—each with its pros and cons. Since there are so many of them, it's really up to you to find ones you like. Personally, some specific exercises really bug my shoulders (overhead press, I'm looking at you). I should just do them anyways because everyone does those workouts, so they must be good, right? Wrong! Every individual is different, and since there is such a variety of exercises, you can really find ones out there that work for you. That variety means I don't really want to get into specific workouts and how to do them. That'd take forever!

However, what is essential about the exercises that you choose is that you have the proper form. Often, comparing yourself to others and ego can get in the way. "How much can you bench?" among other classic bro statements can make you want to lift as much as possible, regardless of form. Sure, many people find motivation in lifting lots of weight, but it's essential to get the form down first when you're starting out. You should start with almost no weight, and that's fine! Even those gym bros started with lightweight reps and perfected their form. You'll usually find the people who lifted lots of weight with poor form at the chiropractor.

Another essential aspect of resistance training is your breathing technique. You should be breathing consistently and steadily throughout your workouts. I know, sometimes my own intelligence astounds me. Who would think of breathing consistently? While this suggestion might sound like the most obvious thing you've ever heard, often, it actually won't be entirely natural. When you're starting out lifting, you'll have to focus a bit on breathing consistently and not taking big gasps in and out, or worse, not breathing at all. While I'm talking about things that seem obvious, remember to hydrate while you're doing resistance training. After each set, take a small sip of water to maintain hydration without getting bloated.

When deciding on exercises you'd like to do, it's best to go to someone who has done resistance training before. That way, they can ensure you're breathing and have the correct form, at least to start out. If that's not an option, you can search for exercises online. Just be sure to start with very light weights and focus on form in online videos. There's no sense in rushing to lift heavier weight and hurting yourself.

Even while taking smart precautions, injuries can still happen. So what should you do when you feel like you've hurt something? Stop immediately at the first sign of bad pain. I think there's a bit of a learning curve for what kinds of pain are good (muscles burning) and bad. However, if there's any chance you think what you are feeling could be an injury, stop your workout right then. Don't exercise that muscle group and any other muscle groups that may affect it for a few days. Instead, do stretches of the afflicted muscle group in the meantime, and maybe stretch some other muscle groups even while you're at it! If the pain goes away in the following days, try working out that muscle group again, but cautiously. Start at a lightweight and slowly build up to where you were. If the pain does not go away, consider seeing your doctor or a physical therapist. All of these methods will help to prevent a long-term injury.

The last important part about resistance training I'll mention is to track track track! I talked a lot about tracking and writing down your progress in the chapter on committing to making a change. As I mentioned, there are many ways to record your results. You should record things like which workouts you do, the weight you're lifting, and the number of sets and reps you did of each exercise. You can record however you'd like, as long as you can understand it in the future. It is also good to record which workouts were supersets, drop sets, etc. Note if you felt discomfort during an exercise, so you can approach it cautiously next time. If you want to go the extra mile, keep track of which workouts you enjoyed doing and didn't like doing. When you look back at your tracked workouts, it is really fulfilling to see your consistent progress and can be a great motivator.

Honestly, that was a lot more than I had planned to write about workout principles, self-five to me. Even so, there's so much more to learn about resistance training if it interests you. While this chapter gives you an excellent framework of knowledge to start with, a great place to learn more would be from a personal trainer or physiotherapist if it interests you. Resistance training is an exceptional form of exercise. It can be great for cardiovascular health and train muscle imbalances that improve everyday posture, significantly improving quality of life. Oh yeah, and make you totally hot (not that you weren't already).

ii- Other Forms of Exercise

While I went into depth about resistance training because it's what I have the most experience in, it is far from the only option. There are plenty of other forms of exercise if resistance training does not interest you. I'll say this again and again: your healthy lifestyle in the long term hinges on personal enjoyment. With all of these forms of exercise, most of the general principles discussed in the resistance training section are still very important. Remember to always do an active warmup before exercising and ensure you're staying hydrated. After the exercise, take time to cool down and stretch. These steps will reduce your chances of injury in all forms of exercise and likely increase your performance as well!

Many people with joint issues find success with any exercise in the water. In her book, Exercise in Water, Debbie Lawrence explains how water takes the pressure off joints that are usually weight-bearing by reducing the gravitational pull on the body. At the same time, water is denser than air, so there is more resistance behind every movement. This resistance dramatically increases the force you need to generate to move in water, helping to strengthen your muscles. The consistent difficulty of moving in water also means you will have a steadily high heart rate, great for cardiovascular health. There are plenty of general fitness classes you can find in the water. You could also swim laps by yourself, or even play a sport like water polo, so there are many different ways you can enjoy your time in the water.

Another exercise that many find very engaging is finding a sport that interests you. Whether it be baseball, basketball, soccer, hockey—all of these are great for your cardiovascular health. Team sports require others who rely on you to show up, which can motivate many people. Other slower pace sports such as curling and golf are still great forms of exercise as long as you enjoy them and are consistently doing them. If you golf, try walking rather than taking a cart around. Sports seem to build up a large amount of passion around them and have helped many live long-term active lifestyles. For example, my grandpa (60 years my elder) loves to golf and gives me a run for my money in fitness. Go grandpa! If any sports interest you, give them a shot. You might just find your favourite hobby.

Going on walks and/or runs is another excellent form of exercise. Depending on your end goal, you could build up from walks to runs or just stay on walks if you'd prefer. In this case, phone applications can be a great motivator. Just search up a run tracker on your phone's application store, and there will be many. Applications even exist like Zombies, Run! which makes a fun game out of completing runs.

There are plenty of other exercises and healthy hobbies you can incorporate into your life—hiking, skiing/snowboarding, skating, and many others. You can mix and match these different exercises any way you'd like to! The critical part is getting consistent physical activity in.

Exercising – Specific Circumstances

Great. This guy says this book is for fitness for people with disabilities and proceeds to hardly discuss it. Don't worry, there's a method to my madness. Many of the general principles I have discussed apply to everyone, including people with disabilities. This chapter will unpack which general principles apply to people with mobility issues, cardiovascular disease, and neurodegenerative diseases. It will also suggest variations of exercise regimes to get around barriers these people face to overcome their disability.

i- Exercise for People with Mobility Issues

People with mobility issues face barriers from the very beginning when it comes to exercise, and I mean that literally. Active warmups are an essential part of exercise, but many typical warmups involve being up on your feet to elevate your heart rate. But remember, the critical part of warmups is getting your heart rate up and supplying blood to your muscles, not being up on your feet and moving around.

Some warmup exercises only involve the upper body, accommodating people who cannot move their legs or have trouble moving around—arm swings and circles, for example. Try it out, put your arms straight out to the side of your body about 90 degrees and make small circles in the air. Alternatively, you could do large arms swings where you circle your arms in their full range of motion. Doing ten arm circles in each direction can definitely begin to increase your heart rate. You can try out other movements too, such as shoulder rolling. If you can get up and it is safe for you, get up and walk back and forth. A big part is recognizing the extent of your limitations. You should be pushing yourself enough to get your heart rate up but not enough that your workout becomes unsafe. The best way to determine this point is by consulting a healthcare professional or personal trainer. If you want to find an exercise regime that works well for yourself, start out cautiously to discover your limitations.

Resistance training can be a method of fitness for people with mobility issues. As stated earlier, cardio may seem like a challenging barrier to navigate for people with mobility issues. The weight you work against in resistance training increases the intensity of the exercises, so it is a great way to increase your heart rate, which, in turn, benefits cardiovascular health. While mobility issues decrease the number of available exercises, plenty can still apply. Again, focus on what you can do, not what you can't. We also went over some forms of exercise in the general principles of exercise section that are ideal for people with mobility issues.

Limiting rest time between exercises helps keep your heart rate consistently high. One of the best ways to limit rest time is by stringing multiple exercises together before rest. Consequently, supersets, compound sets, and circuits workouts are all ideal for people with mobility issues. AMRAPS and HIIT workouts are also great options to consider. Depending on the nature of your mobility issue, plan the exercises accordingly. That means if your mobility issue is from being overweight, plan exercises that will help you to burn calories (and diet!). If your legs are entirely immobilized, make the entire circuit upper body exercises. Consult a physiotherapist or personal trainer for rehabilitative exercises if you have a leg injury.

If getting up is going to be a challenge for you, plan to group seated exercises together and then put all the weights you plan on using nearby. This setup will reduce the amount of rest between exercises which helps to keep your heart rate up. When working out in a public gym, group exercises that you lift similar weights on together to avoid hogging all the dumbbells. People hate that! As long as you plan ahead and do these workouts with intensity, resistance training can double as cardiovascular exercise for people with mobility issues. It can also strengthen the underlying cause of mobility issues—just make sure you consult a medical professional beforehand.

Water exercise can be excellent for those with mobility issues, depending on the nature of the problem. People with arthritis and other joint issues may especially benefit because the water reduces stress on the joints. Further, water exercise offers an impressive variety of exercises. Suppose you get bored of water fitness classes. In that case, you could transition to water running or swimming laps. There are even aquatic programs specifically for people with mobility issues.

Again, depending on the nature and severity of your mobility issue, there may also be sports leagues for people with mobility issues. This is especially true if you live near to a big city. I quickly found plenty of local sports leagues for seniors and people in wheelchairs near where I live.

There are probably a few of you reading this chapter who are suffering from a mobility issue that I didn't specifically address at all. Hopefully, I conveyed that there are great options for everyone, even if I didn't bring them up. By reading this book, you've already shown that you're willing to do some research to live a more fit lifestyle. You will have to decide what parts of this book apply to you. If you are willing to meet with a healthcare professional like your doctor, they will know people to point you to so you get the help you need. If a consultation is not an option, you're going to have to be careful while finding what works for you.

In this case, a good starting point is to identify your issue and what it means for your next step. For example, suppose the nature of your mobility issues comes from weight. In that case, the general principles of diet I discussed will be vital for your recovery. If you are older and have joint problems, you will want to focus on the exercise portion, such as water exercise, to keep your heart healthy. For those who have lost the use of their legs, resistance training with circuit workouts or wheelchair sports leagues can suffice. There is a solution for everyone out there. That said, it won't be easy. As a result, it can be helpful to develop a supportive network—especially one that you can relate to easily. If you have anyone in your life who has faced a similar situation and overcome it, talk to them. You can also attend support groups or physical disability chat rooms online.

ii- Exercise for People with Cardiovascular Disease (Interview with an Exercise Physiologist)

For this section, I'm going to do something a little different. I will be interviewing my friend, Isaiah Stime, who works at the Heart Fit Clinic in Edmonton, Alberta as an exercise physiologist. The Heart Fit Clinic is a private cardiac rehabilitation and stroke prevention center that helps people figure out their heart issues and find healthier ways to live. His knowledgeable perspective will teach us more about general principles of exercise, especially for people with cardiovascular issues. Enjoy!

Q – What does a day in the life of an exercise physiologist look like?

I – At the Heart Fit Clinic, a very important part of our treatment is exercise and physical activity, and that's what I specialize in. I develop individualized exercise programs based off of an individual's equipment available as well as their physical and mental restrictions. I also run monitored exercise sessions at the clinic and over video calls. Another important aspect of my job is to conduct fitness tests on the treadmill while monitoring ECG, heart rate, oxygen saturation, rate of perceived exhaustion, and symptoms. Monitoring these levels allows us to design a target heart rate that is safe for the individual to exercise for 20+ minutes. That will work the heart enough to get adaptations and make it stronger.

Q – What type of disabilities do your clients typically have?

I – There's a wide variety of disabilities at our clinic, but the ones we get the most of our people who have had heart attacks and strokes or other cardiovascular-related disabilities. There are also people who are diabetic, have chronic obstructive pulmonary diseases (COPD), or other lung issues. Others have brain damage or neurological disorders. Finally, some individuals are just doing this program for more preventative purposes to avoid heart attacks, strokes, or any other adverse heart effects in the future.

Q – How do people end up deciding to come to your clinic—recommendations from a healthcare professional?

I – Because we're a private healthcare clinic, we don't actually have people that get recommended by a doctor. Our clients have typically gone through the public healthcare system but haven't been able to find answers or tackle their healthcare issues.

Q – I talk about defining what fitness means to you in this book. What do you feel is your definition of fitness?

I – Fitness means doing something that can get your heart rate up, whether it's doing some sort of exercise regime or other physical activity like walking or sports. To me, though, the most significant part about fitness is finding something that you enjoy. Fitness isn't a one-time deal. You don't just do something once, and then you're fit. It's ongoing, and you always have to continue doing. It's a lifestyle. You should also set goals for yourself, so you can objectively see some of your long-term progress.

Q – Say there's a powerlifter whose only fitness goals are to lift a bunch of weight. He has done resistance training for years and is extremely strong but neglects cardio and eats lots of unhealthy foods to reach his high-calorie demands. With your definition in mind, would you consider them fit?

I – That's a tricky question because I think being fit is a very subjective term. Even though they may look fit and muscular, what's going on inside may not always be great, so being fit does not necessarily mean you are healthy.

Q – What does a regular exercise regime look like at your clinic?

I – At the clinic, each exercise routine is individualized for that person's specific needs. Each program will look different from the next, but generally, it starts with a consultation. At the consultation, we determine the goals and restrictions to make the program. When we exercise, we begin with an active warmup to ensure that we are getting blood flow to the muscles, loosening muscles and joints, and, crucially, getting the heart rate up. Next, we usually start our clients on high-intensity interval training (HIIT) exercise. The purpose is to train our heart and vessels to recover more effectively because the heart rate will go up and down during this exercise style. Usually, this portion involves weight training and cycles through six to 10 exercises in three rounds. We typically add a cardiovascular piece to the HIIT workout, which generally involves a five-minute warmup working up to a client's target heart rate. After, the client does activities to remain at this heart rate for 20 minutes. Once they finish, they have a five-minute cooldown before stretching. That's usually how we start out for all clients, but if there are individuals who are more fit, we may change the style and difficulty of the program.

Q – Are there any other types of exercise programs that you use frequently?

I – Our other exercise program is referred to as ABCT training, developed by Dr. Mark Houston out in the States. It went through about 20 years of meticulous research and studies with cardiologists and exercise physiologists. The end result was a workout program suitable in a cardiac rehabilitation setting. Five sets help the trainer or exercise physiologist adapt the program to the individual's fitness level. Set one starts with five exercises where the client performs one set of several exercises to 12 repetitions. Afterwards, there are five minutes of interval training on the treadmill or any kind of cardio device. From there, they can continue on to sets two to five, where they continue to add sets or volume to the exercises.

Q – What are the biggest differences between an exercise regime at your clinic verse a regular exercise regime?

I – The biggest difference is the safety aspect—being able to monitor the exercises and tailor the program based on a person's restrictions. Most of the people at the clinic have prior heart conditions or even heart attacks, which means we need to monitor them to ensure that the exercise is safe. Most of them will have a lower target heart rate than most people. Personally, when I exercise, I push myself as hard as possible, but most of our clients require breaks, taking blood pressure between sets, and just going a bit slower overall. Another vital aspect of what we do at the clinic is monitoring symptoms. We need to make sure that exercise is symptom-limited depending on what kind of health condition the individual has so that no adverse things happen.

Q – You mention heart rates being a really important thing to monitor for people with cardiovascular issues. What is a good heart rate target for somebody with cardiovascular issues versus a person without any?

I – Yes, it will change a little bit. It's hard to give you a specific number because it really depends on the individual. We do the exercise treadmill test at the clinic to determine a target heart rate. Often, the target heart rate will be lower in people with cardiovascular issues because their blood pressure gets way too high during exercise. If they get their heart rate too high, their risk of heart attack or stroke increases, and it will also damage the arteries and the lining of the vessels. Generally, for someone without any cardiovascular issues, a good tip is to exercise at about 80% of your heart rate max. A typical heart rate max is 220 beats a minute minus your age. So if you are 55, your heart rate max would be 165. 80% would be 165 multiplied by 0.8, which equals 132 beats a minute. Trying to push your heart rate to this amount is key for developing heart adaptations. Heart rate is a fantastic indicator of your physical activity's difficulty. If you reach a heart rate of 115 in one session and 130 during another, you know the intensity of the second session was better.

Q – You talk about the importance of monitoring an individual with cardiovascular issues for safety. What if money is a barrier to an individual, and they can't afford to go to a specialized clinic?

I – The biggest thing I would do is make sure you are doing exercises that are symptom limiting. Make sure you aren't feeling any symptoms, and if you are, stop or decrease the intensity. Symptoms include shortness of breath, chest tightness, dizziness, or anything like that. When exercising by yourself, it's also important to be safe rather than sorry. Start at a lower intensity level and work yourself up slowly instead of going from no exercise or occasional walks to CrossFit or other super high-intensity exercises. Work up your intensity gradually, and don't work yourself to the absolute maximum to reduce your risk of adverse cardiovascular events.

Q – Do you have any favourite exercises for your clients?

I – While I don't personally have any favourite exercise for my clients, I typically try to include exercises that my clients enjoy. I also ensure that we hit every major muscle group, so I always include a variety of exercises. Often, our clients enjoy certain sports and want to do strength training to get better at that specific activity. If that's the case, I am sure to throw in sport-specific exercises. Usually, the exercises I choose are multi-joint movements, so multiple muscle groups get involved, and I will often put multiple exercises together.

Q – When people look for specific exercises for their routine, is there any advice you would give them?

I – Generally, when you are weight training, you should make sure you are hitting all the major muscle groups at least twice a week, so select your exercises with that objective in mind.

Q – What do you think the best motivators for your clients are?

I – Because we're a private healthcare clinic that specializes in getting people healthier, I usually start by explaining how important exercise is for your health and your heart. For our clients, I think their biggest motivation is wanting to be healthy and complete a lifestyle change that involves more physical activity and exercise. Another major motivator for my clients is goals—whether that's looks, reducing pain from physical injuries, or other typical weight loss and strength goals. So on top of their health goal, they will often also have more general fitness goals. As I've already talked about, the final motivator is enjoyment. If you're doing sports you like as a form of cardio or finding exercises you enjoy doing, it can be a great motivator.

Q – At your clinic, you look for motivators to help drive your clients, but many people try to exercise at home and don't have anyone else helping to motivate them. You personally exercise from home quite frequently. How do you motivate yourself?

I – I am a very goal-driven person, so I like the goal-setting approach. When I set goals, I make sure these are SMART goals, which is an acronym for specific, measurable, attainable, realistic, and time-bound. I also know that I am very sports-motivated, so I often tailer my exercises for sports performance. In addition, I have a passion for fitness which drives me. When attempting to motivate yourself, identify your strengths and use these to your advantage.

Q – How important is taking time aside to plan and track your goals?

I – Planning is really important, especially for resistance training. You should know what you're going to do before going into the gym. This way, you can select exercises specifically tailored to your goal. Track your exercises, including your weights and reps for resistance training and your speed, incline, time, and heart rate if you are on a treadmill. This way, you can see if there is some kind of progressive overload to each exercise. Suppose you are doing the same speed or volume over and over. In that case, you will not get any better or develop any adaptations. Another reason tracking is essential is the motivation you get from seeing your progression. If one month you are benching 125 by six, and next you are benching 145 by six—that minor progression can help you feel like you are on track even if it doesn't feel like you are any stronger or better.

Q – What kind of diets do your clients usually have when they come in, and what do you change about those diets?

I – When clients come into the clinic, we generally start by giving them a five-day food log. For five days, they write down what they're eating for each meal, and from there, we identify where we can tweak and modify their diets. When they come in, clients usually eat a high number of processed foods, frequenting fast-food restaurants multiple times per week. They usually have lots of sugary pop and fruit juices, consume few vegetables, and have high carbohydrates in each meal. Before writing down what they eat, people usually believe they generally eat healthily and have a hard time coming to terms with cutting back on certain types of food. The changes we make include entirely cutting out processed foods, sugars including pops, and increasing the number of vegetables they consume.

Another common thing in the diets of people who come into the clinic is super fatty breakfasts high in starches and simple carbohydrates. The nutritionist at our clinic recommends that everyone add some sort of vegetables to their breakfasts because it's prevalent not to have them. You can get these vegetables in the form of smoothies or foods that aren't even traditionally thought of as breakfast foods. Another tool we can use at the clinic is a green supplement where one scoop is equivalent to 10 servings of greens. As you can see, the right supplements are another great way to ensure you're getting the greens and vitamins that you need.

Another cool thing that we do at the clinic is food sensitivity testing. Food sensitivity isn't necessarily like a peanut allergy or something like that. It's more of an intolerance where food irritates our gut microbiome. The gut microbiome is a collection of different types of bacteria in our gut that are actually really beneficial to us. Upsetting our gut microbiome negatively affects many parts of our body, including our vessels and joints. The worst kind of food sensitivities are what we call "red" food sensitivities. Suppose someone is continually eating foods that are in the red for them. In that case, they may have increased arthritis, bloating, acid reflux and other stomach issues. The food sensitivity test will help us decide which foods should be cut out of people's diets that normally might not be thought of. Dairy is the most common food sensitivity. It's a good bet that cutting back on dairy or using dairy alternatives like oat milk, almond milk, or macadamia milk could benefit most people.

Q – When do you think it is good to work out from home?

I – I think it's good to work out from home anytime. Most people believe that exercise needs to be done in a gym setting, but it can really be done wherever. There are many benefits of home workouts, but the biggest is that they tend to be less time-consuming. With the internet, you can find whatever kind of workout you'd like online too, and exercise bands can be a much cheaper alternative to weights. One of my most significant philosophies regarding fitness is that doing anything is better than doing nothing. If you don't want to commute to the gym or just aren't energized enough to go, that's the best time to do a home workout.

Q - When do you think people should seek out a personal trainer?

Personal trainers work great for people new to exercise who want a program to achieve their goals and are curious about the best techniques and exercises. Many generic programs you can find online are just for general fitness and won't necessarily get you closer to your specific goals. A personal trainer is also great for motivating someone to get to the gym. They'll hold you accountable and ensure you're getting in your sessions for the week. They will also monitor your exercise and make sure your technique is correct so that you're not injuring yourself.

Q – In this book, I discuss people with mobility issues, cardiovascular issues, and neurodegenerative diseases. Are there any other groups you can think of where having a fit lifestyle can be more difficult?

I – I'll share an example of an individual from the clinic. About 15 years ago, he got in a car accident and suffered a brain injury. This affected his life in many different ways. He can't stare at screens or be in light rooms too long, and if he exerts himself too much, it will actually cause some memory loss. He played volleyball once a week, and at times he would forget what happened up to 24 hours before the exercise. It's situations like this where we can help at the clinic. We can start by exercising them while they are being monitored, and we can keep an eye on those symptoms. From there, we will make sure that progression is slow enough that we won't make anything worse and we are exercising safely. Even after a couple of weeks combined with our enhanced external counterpulsation (EECP) therapy, he can work out two or three times per week with us and doesn't experience any of those memory loss symptoms. So there are many different challenges and barriers that can impact people's abilities to exercise. Still, there's almost always a solution that you can find to live a more fit lifestyle.

Q – You talk about there being many barriers for people exercising. Can you expand on that thought?

I – For most people, the top three barriers are motivation, time, and energy. Motivation to do any kind of physical activity is often low. They often say they are too busy with family or other commitments, or after a long day of work, they don't want to exercise or do any physical activity. I've already talked a little bit before about how much finding exercise that you enjoy will help to improve motivation. In addition, we often will hold clients accountable by having video calls or zoom sessions. We will watch their exercises to improve their motivation and accountability and give them tips along the way. Instead of paying people to do it, you could also ask a family member or friend to have a weekly call so they can check in on your exercises.

Time is a tough one because people will often have really long days, and the last thing they want to do with their bit of spare time is to work out. What I'd say is that even just going for a walk is good. As I said, doing anything is better than doing nothing.

You could also try doing HIIT training, and you'll be finished in 20 to 30 minutes.

Another thing that I would suggest is setting a timer for yourself. Say as soon as you get home from work, set a 30-minute timer. After this, you can get a snack and whatever you need, but once that 30 minutes is up, you go and exercise.

As for the energy aspect, finding the time of day that you are most energized will be the best time for you to work out. You'll be more motivated and get a better workout at this time. Make sure that you're getting enough sleep in general as well. If you have good workouts, you may find this even helps with your sleep as you expend lots of energy. Also, you can try to get your exercise in before work so that you won't have to go do a long, exhausting day of work and then have to exercise afterwards. One final thing I'll recommend is exercising at lunch at work, or even going for a walk.

Q – What advice would you give people with disabilities trying to achieve a more fit and healthy lifestyle?

The biggest challenge for people with disabilities is finding exercises that they can do. A recommendation would be to see a personal trainer to show them activities that they can do moving forward. Even if someone doesn't have the money to see a personal trainer twice a week, they could even just go once and get some exercises that they can do. Another issue they may come across is feeling self-conscious in a gym setting. I would recommend finding exercises that they can do outside or at home in this case. Finally, I would say that finding someone who can exercise with you or even just support you is really important.

iii- Exercise for People with Neurodegenerative Diseases

Exercise is hugely beneficial to people with neurodegenerative disease. Once again, referring to the nature article published in 2019 by Liu et al., exercise can be protective against neurodegeneration by slowing its progression. Currently, no neurodegenerative diseases are curable by medication, meaning that slowing down the disease and alleviating its symptoms is vital for a longer, much higher quality of life. Combining medication and exercise to slow the disease's progression can be additive. However, one of the main benefits of exercise is that it leaves you feeling better, contrary to many medications. That is not to say that exercise should replace your medication—that determination is best left to your doctor. However, for these reasons, I think exercise should be undertaken as long as possible for people suffering from a neurodegenerative disease.

So yes, for about the thousandth time in this book, exercise is crucial! Now are certain types of exercise better for certain neurodegenerative diseases? Lots of evidence suggests that the answer is yes. I will go through my findings on Parkinson's, Alzheimer's, and Huntington's disease, but no matter what neurodegenerative disease you have, there are likely exercises that may be particularly beneficial! Conversely, certain exercises may be dangerous for you. For this reason, you should always consult a medical professional to ensure that you will be safe doing a specific exercise regime.

For Parkinson's, the American Parkinson Disease Association (APDA) suggests focusing on four core elements when exercising: aerobics, strengthening, balance, and stretching. Essentially, Aerobic exercise is getting your heart rate up, which you might accomplish using HIIT training or circuits during your resistance training. These forms of exercise will fulfill both the elements of strengthening and aerobics. If you don't like those options, you could do brisk walks or runs and band resistance training instead. For balance, APDA suggests tai chi or dance, but if you have no interest in these, that's okay! There are plenty of exercises that train balance. Most involve being on one leg or inexpensive equipment like yoga balls. For stretching, they suggest yoga, but you could also look up your own stretches. The important thing is to stretch your whole body so your entire body gains flexibility and avoids imbalances. Further, the APDA references a study that suggests aerobic activity may be extra beneficial for Parkinson's patients. Turns out, high-intensity exercise resulted in less loss of motor function than both low-intensity exercise and no exercise.

The United Kingdom's leading dementia charity, the Alzheimer's Society, has several suggestions for people with Alzheimer's in the early and middle stages of dementia. For those who don't know, dementia is a decline in cognitive function, including memory, reasoning, and critical thinking. While there are many underlying causes of dementia, Alzheimer's is the most common. So while the exercises are great for people with Alzheimer's, they can apply to many others as well. People with dementia should get at least 150 minutes per week of exercise. In the early and middle stages of dementia, you can refer to many of the activities I covered throughout the chapter on the basic principles of exercise. Continue to do what you enjoy the most and comes easy to you. In the later stages of dementia, the exercises are vital for maintaining your strength and flexibility, though they are dialled back. For example, the Alzheimer Society recommends activities such as shuffling along the edge of your bed in a seated position. This activity may seem really simple, but it will help maintain strength in your muscles responsible for standing from a chair, so it's an important exercise! They also suggest balancing in a standing position and sitting unsupported, without any backrest. It is essential that when someone does these exercises in the later stages of dementia, they are supervised so they don't hurt themselves.

The Huntington's Disease Association (HDA), another United Kingdom charity, stresses the importance of exercise in the early stages of Huntington's disease to maintain quality of life. In what has become a running theme throughout this book, the organization recommends visiting a physiotherapist specializing in Huntington's disease to develop an ideal fitness routine. The HDA's fitness program includes flexibility training, especially for the trunk (chest, abdomen, pelvis, and back), aerobic training, balance, and strength training. Again, multiple aspects, such as aerobic and strength training, can be combined into a single routine.

Among the many benefits of exercise for people with neurodegenerative diseases, the most amazing one is empowering people to help themselves in a situation where they may feel powerless. While barriers can impact people with mobility issues, cardiovascular disease, neurodegenerative disease, or other disabilities, there is usually a way to stay fit. Given the numerous health benefits, finding a regime that works for you is well worth the effort. And as always, if it is in any way possible, consult a healthcare professional about the exercise you would like to undertake. They'll have the expertise to keep you safer!

Starting your Exercise Program

How do you get started finding an exercise routine that will work best for you? Will you prefer exercising from home or in a public space? How do you know if you're interested in a particular exercise program? The answer to all of these questions is the exact same. Go out there, see what is around you, and try it out! In this chapter, I'll suggest where you can get started with the various forms of exercise I've discussed.

i- Resistance Training at the Gym

Let's start out by discussing resistance training. As always, if you have a disability that may affect your safety while exercising, you should start by talking to a healthcare professional. An excellent option for many people is seeing a physical therapist. Physical therapists have extensive knowledge of exercising correctly and adapting exercises to fit your specific needs. There are physical therapists who specialize in everything from sports to geriatrics. If you ask your doctor about seeing a physical therapist, they will help you find one with a specialty relevant to your situation. Physical therapists will not only increase the safety of your exercises, but they will also help you get to your fitness goals quickly.

If you aren't dealing with any kind of disability or physical therapy is not an option, another good way to start is seeing a personal trainer. While they are not required to have the copious amount of schooling as physical therapists, they often have a wealth of knowledge of exercise routines. Personal trainers deal with many beginners, teaching them the ropes of resistance training as well as advanced techniques when they're ready. Not only will they create a routine for you to reach your goals, but they will also ensure your form is up to snuff and that you are pushing yourself. For some people, personal trainers are a great option long-term because they motivate them to continue exercising. If money is an obstacle for you, but you like the idea of going to a personal trainer, there are alternative options. As Isaiah briefly mentioned in his interview, you could hire a personal trainer for a few months to start off and learn from them and then stop training with them after that to save money. You'll have to decide for yourself if you will be able to motivate yourself if you no longer have a personal trainer. I know many people who have spent money on personal trainers, and it worked really well for them. They got really fit while they had their personal trainer but lost all momentum after going it alone. If you intend to transition away from a personal trainer, keep in mind you will need to find ways to motivate yourself afterwards.

Finally, if you're an adamant do-it-yourself person like I am, or money is a barrier, these strategies are effective ways to start up at the gym. Many people find it intimidating to go to a gym when you're starting out. Who wants the scrutinizing gaze of seasoned Chads that have been going to the gym for years? While in actuality, this kind of alpha-bro judgement hardly ever happens because everyone is so focused on themselves, the anxiety many people feel is entirely normal. There are a few solutions that will help you feel more prepared for the gym.

One option is to start resistance training with somebody you know who has lots of experience. Have them take you through a few workouts and evaluate your form, and don't be afraid to ask questions! After a few workouts, you'll probably feel a whole lot more prepared to go it alone. That said, workout partners can be a great form of motivation, as you both drive each other to keep going. I've talked about getting a workout partner who is experienced, but any partner from beginner to experienced can help motivate you. However, one potential issue is missing workouts because you're both not available, making it more challenging to turn exercising into a habit. Plan ahead by making a consistent workout schedule with your partner to avoid this hangup. If one of you is not available for a workout, continue with the regular workout schedule without them for a day if possible. Consistency is key for turning working out into a habit!

Another option is to do research by yourself to start out. This option is less safe than the others I have suggested so far but is considerably better than just wandering into a gym with no plan. As I talked about, planning your workouts is critical. There are many workout routines you can find online. Personally, I would search "beginner push day workout" online. There will be many potential options, but take the time to look up and understand all the exercise forms in the workout plans you are interested in. Videos are often beneficial to learn forms correctly since these exercises are all motion-based. Once you've found an option that works for you, record the workouts and go to the gym. Start out at very light weights until you've perfected the form of an exercise before pushing yourself to reduce your chance of injury.

ii- Resistance Training from Home

What if people don't have access to a gym or don't want to go but are still interested in resistance training? For these people, working out from home may be a good option. Home workouts are also ideal when you have limited time or energy. It doesn't take long to get an effective workout in—even as few as 20 minutes! That means, for many people, commuting to the gym can take even longer than the exercise. By exercising at home, you save this time and don't expend unnecessary energy getting to the gym. With a bit of creativity, doing resistance training from home can be inexpensive with the right supplies. One of the cheapest options is to purchase some resistance bands and cables. You can get a complete set of resistance bands and cables for around $30 or cheaper if you get them used. These are really versatile tools that can enable you to do many different exercises. With resistance bands, cables, and bodyweight exercises, you should get a complete workout that works great for beginners. If you work out from home, the principle of researching your workouts is even more vital. There won't be any gym staff trained in first aid in your garage! Great form and knowing your limits will keep you safe at home.

If you want to gain muscle or have more advanced workouts, dumbbells and a bench are a good step up beyond the resistance bands and cables. You can find new adjustable benches for about $150, and dumbbells cost about $2/lb, so this isn't a particularly cheap option! The adjustable bench will be crucial to work your muscles from multiple angles. Adjustable dumbbells are another great option if you can lift lots of weight. You can find them for about $300 each. They usually go from about 5 to 90 lbs with 5 lb increments. With cables, a bench, and dumbbells, you should be able to do a great full-body workout from home, even if you are at a more advanced fitness level.

iii- Other Forms of Exercise

This section will focus on the general fitness programs I discussed earlier, including running, water exercise, and sports programs. Something to consider is that the programs available to you will vary depending on where you live. I'll present different strategies to find these programs and demonstrate how to use them by finding programs near me in Edmonton, Alberta.

If water exercise interests you and you have a pool near where you live, it is a great fitness opportunity. Even if you don't know how to swim, if you ask about swimming lessons at your local pool, they are likely to have a program you could attend. If your local pool does not have lessons, try searching for swimming lessons online instead. Most swimming programs are relatively affordable and a great source of exercise. Unfortunately, with COVID, these lessons are less widely available. You may have to look around or even wait until they are available again. If you already know how to swim, exercise can be as simple as going to your pool a few times a week and swimming around. Depending on your fitness level, you could swim laps, just tread water, or do some water running. Whatever you choose is up to you! The important part is that the activity should push you enough to increase your heart rate. Swimming around the pool is a wonderful option if you are self-motivated.

If you are not as self-motivated, I'd suggest enrolling in programs that involve other people. One option is enrolling in an aquacise class. Aquacise classes are usually offered at larger pools, which you can usually find online. In Edmonton, the Scona pool offers an aquacise class included in the pool's monthly and annual pass fees, so it's very affordable! If you enjoy sports, try out water polo if you can! Unfortunately, water polo is less widely available to the general public. In Edmonton, if you are a University of Alberta student, there is a water polo club made for beginners and advanced players. There is also a water polo club for kids. Finding places to play water polo will be more challenging if you are not in one of these age ranges. In lieu of any local programs, you could ask some friends to play water polo with you. An added benefit here is the motivation that friends can provide for exercise.

Another thing that may have interested you is sports leagues. Many sports are widely available to all age groups at local recreation centres. Sports offer a great combination of social interaction and fitness motivation that makes them unique. People often find they are passionate about sports which makes it an ideal form of fitness. Financially, there is a significant difference between different sports leagues because of the equipment involved. Basketball, soccer, volleyball, and baseball are more affordable, while something like hockey is a bit more expensive. Depending on how much you've played the sport and your competitiveness, there are different leagues to play in. For example, there are sports and social clubs like the Edmonton Sports and Social Club. These offer sports programs mainly for beginners who casually play the games. Despite the casual nature of these games, they still make for great exercise. It focuses on the social aspect of getting out there and playing with some teammates in friendly games.

There are also men's, women's and co-ed leagues that are far more competitive. If you love competition but are a beginner, this could still be an excellent option for you. These programs often have different tiers for multiple skill levels. High-tier leagues usually have practices and very talented players, great for people with lots of experience who want to put extra time into the sport. Low-tier leagues are still competitive but usually have less skillful players, and many teams don't have practice times. These commitments will vary from team to team, but that is the general trend. It is really fortunate that a large amount of people enjoy sports because there are so many people in these leagues that a good option is usually available to everyone. Competitive people who play at a high level, people who play at a high level but just want to play casually, inexperienced players... the list goes on. There is a league for everyone so you can have judgment-free fun. Just read about the league you are going into, and you should find the level of skill and competitiveness perfect for you.

Going on walks and runs is another excellent way to stay fit and can be done virtually anywhere. Walking is fantastic for beginners who believe that other forms of exercise are too intense for them. Even 10 minutes of walking can be really impactful in changing sedentary lifestyles. Walks are enjoyable because you can pick whichever environment suits you. If you just want a quick walk, just go outside and walk around your house. If there are nice walking paths around your home, even better! There are also plenty of parks that offer beautiful walking paths you could consider. When it is really cold or hot out, gyms will often have tracks where you can walk laps around too. Walks and runs are obviously very self-motivated routes. Still, there are a few tricks if you are not self-motivated.

One idea is to get a walking buddy to improve motivation and just enjoy their company. One method I've personally found really successful is going on walks with my dog. If you have a dog like mine, a walking addict, they will drive you to get out and walk, even on days you don't feel like it. Countless times I sat at my desk, in a state of grogginess with no intention of moving. This laziness all changes when I feel the stare of a cute, tiny creature, and begrudgingly I step outside to take a walk. The funniest thing happens when you're out there, walking in the fresh air, seeing your dog enjoy themself. You begin to enjoy yourself as well. I really found that going on daily walks with my dog has been a great form of fitness and is both calming and enjoyable. Keep in mind that while walking is a good starting point, you will ideally need an activity that drives your heart rate up more if you want to continue to improve your fitness. A natural progression of walks is running. You do them in the same places, outside, gym tracks, treadmills, and more. Like I said earlier, there are plenty of running apps that can track your run times which I found really motivating. One thing to note is that running on rough concrete can be pretty hard on your joints. To reduce the wear and tear on your joints, ensure you take short strides and keep your knees low.

Running and walking groups can be perfect if you want to run with more of a social element. You can do this by talking to friends and family about meeting up once a week to go on a walk or run. However, if you cannot muster up enough people, other running and walking groups are available. For example, the Edmonton Running Room offers running clubs, and other running clubs similar to this one are widely available. Consequently, you can turn your exercise into a new hobby while meeting new friends.

If you are a person who enjoys sightseeing, take up hiking and go out there and explore! Start with nearby areas or even go across the globe and see some of the beauty it offers. This is a cheap hobby that is friendly to everyone—from beginners to very fit people. There are reviews of trails online, and if you read into them, you can find out how difficult they are. Many sites even offer a number rating for the difficulty of trails, making it quick and easy to find out. My partner and I had only ourselves to blame as we retreated down a mountain described in one of these reviews as "extremely difficult to hike" in defeat. Another hobby you could take up is skiing and snowboarding if you live in a colder climate. Why else would anyone live in this frozen wasteland we call Edmonton?

While I've only listed a few activities here, there are plenty of other active hobbies that can improve your fitness. Not all of your hobbies need to be fitness-related. In fact, I think having a variety of hobbies is fantastic. If you can at least find one fitness-related hobby that you enjoy, though, it can change your life. With so many incredible opportunities, you really don't have to go far to find a fitness program that works for you.

Interview with a Success Story

"One day, I just woke up and not only did I know that I could get better, I had the absolute knowledge that I would get better, and I just started that day, one thing at a time." - Catherine Mardon

You've now read a lot of advice about committing to making a change, principles of diet and exercise, and finding out what works for you. In this chapter, you'll read about a success story, or as she'd refer to herself, a work in progress. I'll be interviewing Catherine Mardon—writer, social activist, and former lawyer. She had mobility issues due to extremely high weight but has changed her lifestyle to lose much of it. I've discussed a lot about consistency and its importance when you're trying to make a lifestyle change to be more fit. In this chapter, you may notice that I'll depart from my own rules as this interview format will be a little different from the one earlier in the book with Isaiah Stime. Learn from what I write, not what I do.

i- Catherine Mardon

Everyone's situation is unique. To fully understand Catherine's disability, you need to know about the person she is and how her situation affected her mentally. "I played sports when I was younger and had many fairly serious sports-related injuries. I had an ankle that was reconstructed because I tore a bunch of ligaments out; I had several knee surgeries because I tore my ACL, MCL, and cartilage in my knee. The big one, though, was a burst fracture, which basically means I burst the vertebrae at the bottom of the spinal column and the lumbar vertebrae together. That did a lot of damage to the nerves in there. I was unable to move for seven weeks and then spent eight years in a wheelchair, basically having to teach myself how to walk again. Going from being an active person to suddenly very inactive brought on a depression common in great change like that. I self-medicated my emotions and pain through food. The result was gaining an enormous amount of weight after having my back broken."

ii- Catherine on Exercise

Catherine and I went on to discuss exercise for overweight people. She started off by describing common mistakes for overweight people, emphasizing the importance of some of the principles I discussed earlier in the book. "The biggest issue that comes up with many of my overweight friends is that they will get themselves injured. I had a lot of experience with exercise playing sports in the past, but many overweight people never got that kind of experience, so they don't know about the importance of things like warmups and stretches. Even if they try to do it, they don't do it right or long enough, and they get hurt. This can really throw a wrench into their fitness, especially if they need something like surgery."

Next, with injuries in mind, I asked what would be a good starting exercise for someone who is very overweight or obese. "The best exercise for someone who is severely obese is the pool, either walking in the water or water aerobics. Water walking aerobics is great because you can go at your own pace, and you don't have the same weight jarring forces on the joints. Even if they've never done any kind of exercise, their joints can be worn out just from carrying that weight around."

Although water aerobics are great for people who are severely overweight, Catherine explained how sometimes the equipment and facilities are not designed for them. "The biggest issue [overweight people] have is finding places to buy swimsuits that fit. There's no place that you can go to locally to try on a swimsuit or any other kind of exercise equipment. You are beginning to see entrepreneurial women making plus-size clothing for outdoor activities like biking, climbing, and hiking. However, clothes for these activities were never designed for larger women. Another issue is finding a handicap-accessible pool. Londonderry pool here in Edmonton is a good example. The leisure pool is handicap accessible, but the lap pool is not. You'd have to get in the leisure side and swim across the entire area to get into the lap area. Not all pools have handicap-accessible changerooms either. If you need an attendant, like in my case my husband, then they can't come in with you unless it is in the family room."

Catherine also stresses the importance of having handicap-friendly showers at these facilities,
saying, "for some people who are disabled or overweight, the showers at their local recreation centers are the only ones that they have access to. They often live in apartments that they can't use the shower at."

This lack of equipment and facilities for obese people extends beyond the pool. Catherine explained,
"exercise equipment has weight limits a lot of the time. Even if you find an exercise bike that can handle your weight, it is often so uncomfortable you can't ride it for any length of time."

While these limitations may seem intimidating, Catherine found many different ways to make exercise comfier for herself. She related, "my exercise bike had a Hobson easy seat. It's a two-cheek seat that is adjustable, so you can have it on your butt cheeks rather than in between them. These seats are much more comfortable. Another thing that will make you less likely to be hurt is comfortable running/exercise shoes. Finally, the last thing I'll recommend to newbies is a hand crank bike. You can put it on the coffee table and use your hands or put it on the floor in front of your favourite chair and use your feet. It can be both an upper or lower-body workout. You can get them for $100 on Amazon. Even somebody who is in a studio apartment would have room for this. It's perfect for people who have weight-bearing limitations."

Not all the barriers facing overweight people from fit lifestyles are physical. Others are psychological or emotional. Catherine reasoned, "one thing that discourages overweight people from attending water aerobics classes is not wanting to be next to all the skinny people. I always tell them, don't worry about it. The water aerobics classes have many old people, people rehabilitating injuries, and fat people. If you're afraid you're going to be outshined by a hardbody, they're all upstairs in the gym trying to attract the cute guys."

She finished by discussing common pitfalls for people who try water aerobics, "another thing that my friends talk about is trying to get exercise buddies. 90% of the time, their exercise buddy bugs out, though. My roommate wanted to come with me to water classes and came along a couple of times, but she had chronic obstructive pulmonary disease and couldn't breathe well in the water, so she quit and kind of wanted me to quit too. You have to get into the mindset that you're doing this for yourself. I told myself that I'm responsible for everything I do. I'm responsible for getting myself to pool, I'm responsible for getting myself to the gym, I'm responsible for getting myself to the nutritionist, I'm responsible for everything that I eat."

There are plenty of disabilities that can add additional barriers to someone's fitness journey. Catherine notes, "One group that you don't cover in your book is people with congenital issues. Some kids with fetal alcohol syndrome don't have properly developed bones. They don't weight bear correctly, so they can't do things like weight lifting or jumping jacks. Their exercise will have to be things like biking, swimming, or the hand crank bike that I talked about. There are going to be limits. Another thing to consider is when people are nearly or completely bed-bound. When I was close to that, I started with sit-ups and scissor kicks. After that, I started watching exercise videos making the motions while lying on the bed. So I'd do things like jumping jacks just using the arms and legs. It's non-load bearing but completely aerobic, so activities like this would also apply to people with load-bearing congenital issues. After a while, I graduated to doing these exercises on a chair. They have chair aerobics, but they're usually designed for older people who are arthritic and want to increase their mobility. If you have someone who is 600 pounds, they will need an aerobic workout that's a little higher intensity.

So following these fitness workouts is a good way that I found to increase the intensity without injuring myself."

Exercise, however, is only part of living a fit and healthy lifestyle, something that Catherine believes is not well understood. "When I began to exercise again, exercise alone probably did not lose me a single pound. That's a misnomer many people have—they think they can lose weight only with exercise, and you can't. Losing one pound of weight is approximately 3500 calories, and burning that much with exercise is nearly impossible. One thing we tell a lot of newbies is that you exercise for mobility, some muscle building (which can burn calories), and for endorphins. Don't expect to lose weight exercising."

"If you want to lose weight, any diet that restricts calories can do it for you. The first part is calorie in, calorie out, period. However, the second part comes to exercise, and it can be looked at in terms of convenience and desirability. If there's something you really like to do, you will do whatever it takes, even if it takes a long time to get there. If it's an exercise you hate, it has to be something you can roll out of bed and do in five minutes. You have to find exercises with the right combination of convenience and enjoyment that you will actually do it. I found running in chest-deep water really therapeutic because that basically put me at the weight I was the last time I ran. I felt like a 25-year-old. It was wonderful. There were times I would get up at 4:30 AM to go to the pool while it was -40 °C out, so if you find something you really enjoy, it doesn't have to be as convenient, and you're more likely to do it."

iii- Catherine on Diet

We then switched our focus from exercise to diet. Catherine relates, "I viewed the diet side of it as a bank. I had gotten myself in debt x number of calories, with each pound I wanted to lose being about 3500 calories. I had to pay myself back, 1 calorie at a time. I could not think about how I wish I could have started 10 years ago, or I wish I could go back to my 16-year-old self and warn about letting it get this bad."

She then described a fascinating analogy to drive home the importance of being realistic with yourself and taking it one step at a time. "Teddy Roosevelt Jr., his dad was president of the United States, he was in the army. On D-Day in World War II, he was the highest-ranking general that went onshore in the first wave. For weeks, they practiced how they would attack Utah Beach in France. They had everything set up, including bombing the area beforehand to prepare for their arrival. When they got onto shore off their boats, they realized they were not on Utah Beach at all. Teddy's officers asked him how their reinforcements would find them and if they should get back in the boats and go back to the correct beach. Teddy replied that this may not be the beach they planned for but that their war started here. Teddy went on to win the medal of honour that day. Being extremely overweight was really not the beach that I ever expected to end up on. It isn't the beach I wanted to be on, but it's the beach I was on, and I committed to starting the war from here. That's the mindset that many successful people get on to. You can't beat yourself up for what you did. You just have to start from where you are."

So Catherine started right from there with dieting and mimicking the motions of exercise videos in bed.

Catherine's mindset continued over time, where she tried out many different types of diets with her husband, Austin. "My husband has lost 50 lb on Jenny Craig, and I had lost 80 lb before a lymphedema problem I developed. I've also lost weight on the Atkins keto diet, Nutrisystem, and Weight Watchers. The diets that have worked best for me are diets where I don't have to think, including Nutrisystem and Jenny Craig because they had pre-made meals. When I was on my way home from work, it was nice having a meal that I knew would be ready to make, and it stopped me from getting takeout after a long day at work. The most important thing is something you can stick to."

"When I lost the most weight, I ate the same things for breakfast, lunch, and dinner. For breakfast, I had cheerios and yogurt. I had a veggie burger on pita bread for lunch, and for dinner, I had vegetables and chicken breast. That would drive most people crazy, but it worked great for me. I am a hardcore food addict. Me being in the kitchen is the same as being an alcoholic working as a bartender. That's another reason why Jenny Craig works great for me. I can't allow myself to start cooking because I am a great cook with an excessive love for food. Jenny Craig gives me the pre-made meals so I won't go overboard. I've even channelled my love for cooking in spices instead of the substance of the meal itself. I'm eating these small meals with Greek oregano on them or bass-smoked paprika, so that's how I've channelled my love for food. It's a tiger—you can only tame it; you can't kill it!"

iv- The Mind Games

Catherine has made substantial changes to her life from the beginning of her journey. What made her commit to making this kind of change? Catherine explains, "You really do get to a point where you give up. I had been taking care of other people and their kids, basically everyone except myself. This may not make a lot of sense, but one day I just woke up and not only did I know that I could get better, I had the absolute knowledge that I would get better, and I just started that day, one thing at a time."

"You can pray for a miracle to get healed or skinny, but I didn't get that miracle. I got the miracle of my spirit getting healed rather than my body; I had to take care of that myself. I had a gazillion wake-up calls while I was gaining weight. The first time I couldn't buy clothes at a store, that would've clued many people in. I didn't, though. I sew, so I just made my own. Every time I needed new pants, I just added a few inches to the pattern. I also ended up in the hospital with an angina attack. They couldn't diagnose me because I was too large to have an angiogram. The only thing they could properly measure was that I had high blood pressure. The cardiologist even sent me home saying that my character was too flawed for him to help. He sent me home with only a bunch of blood pressure medication, basically to die. Many different things could've been causing the angina pain, but fortunately for me, it was actually the blood pressure, and I survived. I should've had a trashed heart and liver, but I was lucky and didn't. This ultimately resulted in me needing to take nitroglycerine six times a day. Even this only persuaded me to lose weight for a little while."

Catherine explained that committing to change and continuing that habit can be complicated. "If near-death didn't do it for me, I truthfully don't know exactly what it was. I also do therapy for emotional eating because I have PTSD. There I learned other methods to deal with it besides eating. Sometimes I have success with this, and sometimes I don't. It's something I can contain but never conquer, you know—that thing in my head that tells me to have ice cream when I have a bad day."

With this in mind, I asked Catherine if she had any advice for other people trying to make that first step to live a more fit life. She answered, "For most people, I'm sure it would help to write down the things that they would like to do and can't, like a bucket list."

While you should have fitness goals to shoot for, Catherine explained the importance of still living your life, no matter what weight you are. "One of the things that overweight people often do is say that as soon as they lose weight, they will do this or that. We literally waste huge hunks of our lives waiting to live once we lose weight. It's really important to live even while you have that weight. If you want to go to a ball, just buy a big ball gown. You don't have to wait until you lose weight to buy a smaller one. If you buy nice clothes and feel better about yourself then lose weight, it's okay. Many overweight people sit there in terrible clothes. They feel awful about themselves because they don't want to spend money on good clothes until they lose weight. I went ahead and bought myself nice clothes, then felt really good about myself, then lost weight. Just do baby steps. It can take six weeks to six months for a new habit to form."

This brings an interesting point up—confidence in oneself is critical because if you are confident, you are more likely to take that first step. So in a way, taking those steps and building up your confidence at first is the beginning of people's fit and healthy lifestyles.

So after Catherine had taken her first step, I asked her what she did to continue to motivate herself. "When it worked the best, and I'm still a work in progress, was when I didn't think about it. Every time I stopped to think, oh, I've got to do this or that this week, I wouldn't get to exercise. So I stopped thinking. I had a checklist like a pilot would before takeoff, and I wouldn't think. I just went down the list and did. The next thing I knew, I'd be pulling into the parking lot of the YMCA. If I sat and thought about it, I'd be thinking about all the things I had to do when I got home, or that once I got home, I would be tired and wouldn't feel like exercising. I couldn't think about motivation, why I was doing it, or how much I was doing it. I just did."

Motivation in the long-term can be challenging, so I asked Catherine if she had advice for people trying to make a long-term change to their fitness. To that, she said, "You have to keep in mind that you'll only fail if you quit. If you haven't done something for a couple of days or weeks, it doesn't mean that you failed, and it's the end. It may mean that you simply need to start again. You know, forgive yourself. One thing that I've found in many of my overweight friends is that we're a perfectionistic bunch and have many issues with the scale. If I got on the scale and it was one pound more than I thought it would be, I would think it was all over, and I would give up. If I was one pound under what I thought I would be, I would go, wow, I've succeeded, I'm going back to eating like a normal person."

Catherine then reasoned that continuing long-term healthy habits may be even more vital for people who have been overweight. "When you lose a bunch of weight, it will still significantly alter your baseline metabolic rate. If you're the same height and weight as somebody who has been yo-yo dieting, as in constantly going up and down in weight, you may be burning 2000 calories a day while they burn only 1700 calories per day. For the rest of your life, if you've been heavy, you may need to be on a lower calorie count than somebody who hasn't, and you know what, it's not fair. It is what it is though. It's not fair for people who are type one diabetics that have to be on insulin the rest of their life. There are lots of things that aren't fair. Some people are overweight just because of genetics. I genetically am tall and have really big feet, so you know what? I'm not going to be a horse jockey. I'm not going to be a gymnast, and that's not fair either because I was pretty sure I was going to be the next Nadia Comăneci growing up. Still, genetically that wasn't in store for me."

"In our minds, people often think that a pound of fat looks like a pound of butter, but it's not. I had a nutritionist that had a correct anatomical pound of fat, and it's full of blood vessels. If you've ever trimmed dog nails and gone too far, you can hit the blood vessel, and it bleeds. What you have to do is cut up near to it, then that vein will retreat, and in a week, you can trim them a little bit shorter. When you lose weight, that's what happens. The fat that burns first is the fat close to the veins because that's most accessible. Sometimes you won't lose your belly because this fat is being burned first. The veins that grew in your fat all the way to your stomach are still there for this first bit, and the fat cells stay too; they simply get smaller. That's why people who have lost weight can grow it back so quickly. They already developed the veins to support the fat cells in the past, and it is much easier for these fat cells to re-establish themselves.

There is light at the end of this tunnel, though, for people who can continue their healthy habits. "The National Weight Control Registry keeps a registry of Americans who have lost at least 30 lbs and maintained that weight for at least a year. They've found that if you keep the weight off for three years, you have reset your body's natural weight to a lower place. Just like the dog's nails, the veins have reabsorbed in, and it will make it easier to keep off weight. Personally, after keeping the weight off for three years, I've found that at points where I have begun to put on weight again, there was a weight I would stop at that was much lower than my previous high weight. If you can refrain from going back to your high weight within these three years, your chances of going back to your highest weight are greatly diminished."

v- Keep it Light-Hearted

Everyone's fitness journey is different, and often times it's not going to be easy, but it's absolutely possible. Catherine has successfully lost weight and went from not walking at all to walking and swimming comfortably again. Something I noticed about Catherine was that even though her fitness journey was difficult and still continues to this day, she was very light-hearted and had a great sense of humour about it. She even told me, "I'm going to have to wear some support things on my legs, and I got to choose between black or beige. I chose the black ones because then if someone actually sees them, I can say I'm actually cat women, and this is my cat woman suit under my clothes."

Catherine's light-heartedness is infectious and something that, I think, would help anyone to achieve their fitness goals.

Take that First Step, and the Next one…

Let's have a quick recap of everything we've learned from this book. I started out by wasting your time ranting about pierogis. Nice. To be fair, after that, I contained myself pretty well!

First and foremost, you defined what fitness meant to you. While this may have seemed relatively unimportant, it was a vital part of your fitness journey. Without any definition of fitness guiding you, you would have no way to set goals that would get you objectively closer to what you consider fit. Hopefully, you listened to my advice and incorporated being healthy into your definition.

Next, I described three general categories for physical disabilities: mobility issues, cardiovascular disease, and neurodegenerative diseases. Understanding them is key whether you currently struggle, have struggled, or have not dealt with them all in the past. Comprehending these conditions can either help you directly or allow you to learn what these people go through and sympathize with the difficulties they may face.

With those definitions out of the way, we talked about committing to making a positive change in your fitness. Of course, while taking this first step is what I consider the most challenging, it is useless if you do not continue to form a habit that you enjoy. To ensure we achieve this goal, we discussed ways of motivating yourself, forgiving yourself, and picking it back up when you fall off the wagon.

We then discussed what I think to be two crucial components of any healthy definition of fitness: dieting and exercise. Remember to choose options that you enjoy so you are more likely to continue them long-term. We started by talking about general principles for everyone and then transitioned to discussing dieting and exercise specifics for people with disabilities. We learned a lot from Isaiah Stime, an exercise physiologist, during these chapters. Not only did he discuss exercise for people with cardiovascular issues at his cardiac rehabilitation clinic, but he also shared knowledge on exercising and dieting in general.

Next, we considered how to find an exercise routine that works best for us. While specific forms of exercise may stand out to us, the best way to find what works for you is to get out there and try it. We then explored where you could start different forms of exercise to give them a fair try.

Finally, we put it all together and heard from a success story, Catherine Mardon. Her example cements that it is possible to change your lifestyle and be fit, no matter what circumstances you are going through.

I'm not going to claim that this book has everything you need to know to live a fit lifestyle or that it should be easy after reading it. What I hope that you realize from reading this book is that it is possible. You have access to tools around you that could help. You just need to take that first step. Well, actually, the jokes on you. I consider having read this book to be that elusive first step you've been trying to make. It's all out of the way. So, where do you go from here? Spoiler, it's the exact same whether you have a disability or don't.

You continue to progress, write down SMART goals for yourself, and then figure out objective steps you can take to get closer to that. Nobody knows you quite like yourself. Find ways to get motivated and continue. Fail, and then step right back and try again. Live your life, love yourself. One thing being fit won't change is that you're still you, and that's pretty awesome.

Chapter by Chapter References

Fitness with Disabilities

Durães, F., Pinto, M., & Sousa, E. (2018, May 11). Old Drugs as New Treatments for Neurodegenerative Diseases. National Center for Biotechnology Information. Retrieved November 11, 2021, from https://www.ncbi.nlm.nih.gov/pmc/articles/PMC6027455/#:~:text=Currently%2C%20no%20neurodegenerative%20disease%20is,the%20progression%20of%20the%20disease.

Nature. (n.d.). Neurodegenerative diseases. Retrieved November 11, 2021, from https://www.nature.com/subjects/neurodegenerative-diseases

Liu, Y., Yan, T., Chu, J. M. T., Chen, Y., Dunnett, S., Ho, Y. S., Wong, G. T. C., & Chang, R. C. C. (2019, February 26). The beneficial effects of physical exercise in the brain and related pathophysiological mechanisms in neurodegenerative diseases. Nature. Retrieved November 13, 2021, from https://www.nature.com/articles/s41374-019-0232-y

Parkinson's Foundation. (n.d.). Movement Symptoms. Retrieved November 13, 2021, from https://www.parkinson.org/Understanding-Parkinsons/Movement-Symptoms

General Principles of Diet

Government of Canada. (n.d.). Tips for healthy eating - Canada's Food Guide. Canada Food Guide. Retrieved November 19, 2021, from https://food-guide.canada.ca/en/tips-for-healthy-eating/

Michaels, J. (2021, November 2). Jillian Michaels: "Please Don't Eat More Than One Snack A Day." Women's Health. https://www.womenshealthmag.com/weight-loss/a29390073/jillian-michaels-one-snack-a-day/

Harvard Health. (2019, December 11). The truth about fats: the good, the bad, and the in-between. https://www.health.harvard.edu/staying-healthy/the-truth-about-fats-bad-and-good

The American College of Sports Medicine. (n.d.). Protein intake for optimal muscle maintenance. American College of Sports Medicine. https://www.acsm.org/docs/default-source/files-for-resource-library/protein-intake-for-optimal-muscle-maintenance.pdf

Clark, N. (2019, July 17). The Athlete's Kitchen: Carbs in the News. American College of Sports Medicine. Retrieved December 2, 2021, from https://www.acsm.org/blog-detail/acsm-blog/2019/07/17/carbohydrate-news-athletic-performance

Lawrence, D. (1998). The Complete Guide to Exercise in Water. A&C Black.

Dieting – Specific Circumstances

National Heart, Lung, and Blood Institute. (n.d.). DASH eating plan. Retrieved December 5, 2021, from https://www.nhlbi.nih.gov/education/dash-eating-plan

H, G., & Caunca, M. R. (2018, March 7). Mediterranean diet in preventing neurodegenerative diseases. National Center for Biotechnology Information. Retrieved December 9, 2021, from https://www.ncbi.nlm.nih.gov/pmc/articles/PMC7212497/

General Principles of Exercise

Harvard Health. (2020, July 7). Exercising to relax. Retrieved December 15, 2021, from https://www.health.harvard.edu/staying-healthy/exercising-to-relax

National Heart, Lung, and Blood Institute. (n.d.). Physical Activity and Your Heart. Retrieved January 3, 2022, from https://www.nhlbi.nih.gov/health-topics/physical-activity-and-your-heart

Sands, W. A., Wurth, J. J., & Hewit, J. K. (n.d.). The national strength and conditioning association's (NSCA) basics of strength and conditioning manual. National Strength and Conditioning Association. Retrieved January 7, 2022, from https://www.nsca.com/contentassets/116c55d64e1343d2b264e05aaf158a91/basics_of_strength_and_conditioning_manual.pdf

Government of Canada. (n.d.). Physical activity and healthy eating. Canada Food Guide. Retrieved January 10, 2022, from https://food-guide.canada.ca/en/tips-for-healthy-eating/physical-activity-healthy-eating/

Harvard Health. (2020, July 20). Exercise 101: Don't skip the warmup or cooldown. Retrieved January 11, 2022, from https://www.health.harvard.edu/staying-healthy/exercise-101-dont-skip-the-warm-up-or-cool-down

Exercise – Specific Circumstances

Gilbert, R. (2021, October 26). What types of exercise are best for people with Parkinson's disease? American Parkinson Disease Association. https://www.apdaparkinson.org/article/what-exercise-to-do-with-parkinsons/

Alzheimer's Society. (n.d.). Exercise in the early to middle stages of dementia. Retrieved January 16, 2022, from https://www.alzheimers.org.uk/get-support/daily-living/exercise/early-middle-dementia

Huntington's Disease Association. (n.d.). Living well. Retrieved January 19, 2022, from https://www.hda.org.uk/getting-help/if-youre-at-risk/living-well#:%7E:text=Trunk%20mobility%20%26%20flexibility%20exercises%20(e.g.,Strength%20training%2Fcore%20stability.

www.ingramcontent.com/pod-product-compliance
Lightning Source LLC
Chambersburg PA
CBHW030122170426
43198CB00009B/708